WOMEN'S HEALTH IN THE MAJORITY WORLD: ISSUES AND INITITATIVES

WOMEN'S HEALTH IN THE MAJORITY WORLD: ISSUES AND INITIATIVES

LAURIE ELIT

AND

JEAN CHAMBERLAIN FROESE

EDITORS

Nova Science Publishers, Inc.

New York

NOTICE TO THE READER

The Publisher has taken reasonable care in the preparation of this book, but makes no expressed or implied warranty of any kind and assumes no responsibility for any errors or omissions. No liability is assumed for incidental or consequential damages in connection with or arising out of information contained in this book. The Publisher shall not be liable for any special, consequential, or exemplary damages resulting, in whole or in part, from the readers' use of, or reliance upon, this material.

Independent verification should be sought for any data, advice or recommendations contained in this book. In addition, no responsibility is assumed by the publisher for any injury and/or damage to persons or property arising from any methods, products, instructions, ideas or otherwise contained in this publication.

This publication is designed to provide accurate and authoritative information with regard to the subject matter covered herein. It is sold with the clear understanding that the Publisher is not engaged in rendering legal or any other professional services. If legal or any other expert assistance is required, the services of a competent person should be sought. FROM A DECLARATION OF PARTICIPANTS JOINTLY ADOPTED BY A COMMITTEE OF THE AMERICAN BAR ASSOCIATION AND A COMMITTEE OF PUBLISHERS.

LIBRARY OF CONGRESS CATALOGING-IN-PUBLICATION DATA
Available upon request

ISBN 13 978-1-60021-493-6
ISBN 10 1-60021-493-2

RA
778
.W653
2007

Published by Nova Science Publishers, Inc. ✤ New York

CONTENTS

PREFACE

Women's Health in the Majority World: Issues and Initiatives is an innovative text using didactic information and case studies to address those issues that affect most of the worlds women. The first half of the book focuses on health issues that specifically affect women such as maternal morality, fistulas, and cervical cancer. The second part of the book discusses how agencies such as governments, non-governmental organizations, and professional societies can partner and improve standards for women. By affecting the status of women, the whole family and community ultimately benefit.

Chapter 1 - In the developing or majority world, mothers continue to die from largely preventable causes of maternal death. Each year nearly 529,000 will die and another twenty million women suffer from the non-fatal, but significant complications of pregnancy. These devastating deaths and disabilities are partially attributable to low use of skilled attendants and even lower utilization of modern contraceptive methods along with poor access to quality care. The promotion of women's rights and education along with a trans-disciplinary approach to safe motherhood, play an important role in realizing sustainable and real improvement in the lives of thousands of mothers and their dependent children. These foundational steps continue to be major challenges for communities, governments and international organizations to address.

Chapter 2 - Obstetrical fistulas result from prolonged obstructed labor. Approximately 100,000 new cases occur annually predominantly in the developing world.

In this chapter the author discusses the presenting symptoms, associated conditions, and principles of management. Aspects of treatment and health care team training are reviewed. From the patient's perspective the social ramification are immense. However, this tragic circumstance can become an opportunity for education and rehabilitation for the affected woman.

The current health care resources in the developing world can only manage about 10,000 fistula repairs annually. The importance of preventing this tragedy and making resources available to rehabilitate women with fistulas is needed.

Chapter 3 - Millennium Development Goal number five (MDG-5) sets the target that by 2015, maternal mortality ratio will be reduced three-quarters. This is to be done by increasing the proportion of skilled birth attendants providing care in an enabling environment. However, measuring where we are now, and where we will be in 2015 is extremely difficult, if not impossible, because the majority of the women who die, do so in an area of the world with inadequate surveillance or death registration. Efforts to address the difficulty of counting women who die at home, en route to hospital or once in hospital have had mixed success. Efforts to derive a best guess are commonly used though provide a large error range, making before-and-after comparisons inaccurate. Obstetric service indicators are now proposed as a means of measuring whether or not service is adequate, without the effort of counting the women, but this method has yet to be properly evaluated and there may be limitations when this method is transplanted to different settings. Worldwide, skilled birth attendants play an integral role in not only attaining MDG-5, but ensuring we have the numbers to demonstrate that we have truly arrived. As the increase in skilled birth attendants converges with the hoped for decrease in the maternal mortality ratio, a system of counting has to be in place to ensure that women's lives are being saved.

Chapter 4 - For women, cervical cancer is the second most common cancer worldwide. This is unfortunate given that cervical cancer can be preventable through screening programs. If cervical cancer occurs and is identified early, it can be cured with radical surgery or aggressive chemoradiation.

To review the strategies available to prevent or manage cervical cancer.

We will review the global impact of cervical cancer, methods of primary (ie., vaccination) and secondary prevention (ie., cyotology, visual inspection with acetic acid). The important aspects of a screening program will be discussed. Key principals in treatment and management of end stage disease will be reviewed.

Given that cervical cancer is potentially a preventable disease, global strategies toward assessing vaccines, providing screening programs, making available curative treatment and palliative care must be better implemented.

Chapter 5 - To understand the widespread prevelance of anemia in the developing world and its devastating impact on women and children.

This chapter addresses the prevalence, etiology and consequences of anemia. Treatment options are review. Programs which have been effective in reducing anemia like the MICAH program are discussed in detail. This program is based on the principals of evidence, comprehensive multipronged interventions, and collaborative partnerships with the government, health system and community.

Anemia has devastating consequences for women and children, but comprehensive programs have been shown to decrease the devastation of this disease.

Chapter 6 - This article considers the increasing challenge of the fair allocation of scarce public health care resources by focusing on services for women and girls. It considers different ways of thinking about fairness in health care reform, the role of courts in promoting fairness, and the use of affirmative action measures to remedy health disparities. The health of individuals and populations is shown to be affected by clinical services, the organization and functioning of health systems, and underlying socio-economic determinants. Different theories of justice are addressed that affect assessments of fairness, considering availability, accessibility, acceptability of and accountability for services. The transition in judicial dispositions is traced, from deference to governmental resource allocation decisions to evidence-based scrutiny of governmental observance of constitutional and human rights legal obligations. The appropriate use of affirmative action measures to improve equality in health status is explored, given the increasingly unacceptable disparities in health among subgroups of women within countries.

Chapter 7 - The women of Afghanistan faced one of the worst situations in terms of their near enslavement and violation of rights. The importance of education to reverse this trend will be reviewed.

Eight reasons for the oppression of women such as lack of access to justice and misrepresentation of religion will be reviewed. Nine areas for development such as education and access to reproductive health care will be discussed.

For Afghan women to enter the 21st century as productive and healthy members of society, education will play a pivotal role.

Chapter 8 - Health professionals, including obstetricians and gynaecologists, have a strong tradition of involvement in international women's health initiatives in lower resurce countries. These contributions, often initiated by individual professionals through formal but often-informal collaborations, are the basis of the involvement of the Society of Obstetricians and Gynaecologists of Canada (SOGC) in international women's health.

In 1998, the Society committed to pursue excellence in international women's health and to focus its efforts on promoting universal access to emergency obstetric care, as a means to reduce maternal and newborn mortality and morbidity worldwide. Its areas of expertise include increasing access and quality of maternal and newborn health services, including safer pregnancy and delivery and building capacity of professional associations to assume leadership in the field. Its activities are supported by the professional expertise of its members who volunteer as trainers and technical consultants.

This chapter will provide an overview of the international program of the SOGC. It will explore: (a) the contribution of professional associations in global and national efforts to reduce maternal and newborn mortality and morbidity; (b) the partnership model of the Society and its experience in enhancing capacity of professional associations from lower resource countries to assume leadership in the field of sexual and reproductive health; (c) the value of partnerships between professional associations from higher and lower resource countries for the purpose of building capacity.

Chapter 9 - Nongovernmental organizations (NGOs) are typically value-based organizations that depend, in whole or in part, on charitable donations and voluntary service. Although the NGO sector has become increasingly professionalized over the last two decades, it is generally recognized that principles of altruism and voluntarism still remain key defining characteristics.

In this chapter, various definitions of the NGO will be introduced and discussed, including those offered by the World Bank and theWorld Health Organization. A literature review related to the evolving nature of NGO involvement in advancing women's health in the 20th and 21st centuries also will be undertaken. In the review, the authors emphasize the role of NGOs in health service delivery, health promotion, and policy advocacy related to women's health. They also review the evolving participation of international NGOs in initiating and contributing to global health policy and highlight global trends in NGO involvement in women's health.

The following section envisions a future for NGOs. Important questions related to their role in low-resource settings in the 2lst century are delineated. The chapter then explores the key challenges and opportunities for NGOs to address women's health issues. Key challenges include organizational growth and development, assessing and strengthening performance, sustainability, representation and accountability, politicized foreign assistance, religious fundamentalism and human rights. Key opportunities include collaboration with the private sector, the community and government, and reconfiguring reliance on international assistance. The section offers examples of cutting edge NGOs in action and draws from lessons learned by PATH and other international NGOs. PATH is discussed as an example of a specific NGO model that emphasizes collaboration between governments, local NGOs, civil society, and corporate business communities through institutional partnerships. Examples of specific program outcomes illustrate how this model functions successfully.

Chapter 10 - Stephen Lewis' Address September 24, 2004 at the International Women's and Childrens' Health Conference (IWCH) at the Royal Botanical Gardens, Burlington, Ontario.

IWCH is Sponsored by the Department of Obstetrics and Gynecology and the Degroote School of Medicine at Mcmaster University, and Sisters of St. Joseph Health Care Centre, Hamilton, Ontario, Canada.

Chapter 11 - In this chapter the impact of war on the health of women and children in both phases of the war system is considered. Then we will turn to the efforts of women in ending specific wars, preventing war, and further, bringing about a peace system.

In: Women's Health in the Majority World: Issues and Initiatives   ISBN1-1-60021-493-2
Eds: L. Elit and J. Chamberlain Froese, pp. 1-19   © 2007 Nova Science Publishers, Inc.

Chapter 1

MATERNAL MORTALITY AND MORBIDITY: HISTORY'S ONGOING TRAGEDY

Jean Chamberlain Froese[1]

Department of Obstetrics/Gynecology
McMaster University, Canada
Save the Mothers, Uganda

ABSTRACT

In the developing or majority world, mothers continue to die from largely preventable causes of maternal death. Each year nearly 529,000 will die and another twenty million women suffer from the non-fatal, but significant complications of pregnancy. These devastating deaths and disabilities are partially attributable to low use of skilled attendants and even lower utilization of modern contraceptive methods along with poor access to quality care. The promotion of women's rights and education along with a trans-disciplinary approach to safe motherhood, play an important role in realizing sustainable and real improvement in the lives of thousands of mothers and their dependent children. These foundational steps continue to be major challenges for communities, governments and international organizations to address.

INTRODUCTION: THE WORLD LOOKS ON

The tragedy of maternal death and disability continues to plague the world's family and broader community. Despite numerous international conferences and pledges to improve the health of mothers in the developing world, there is still an estimated 529,000 mothers who die yearly from largely preventable causes of maternal death [1]. In addition, another twenty million women suffer from the non-fatal, but significant complications of pregnancy including anaemia, infertility, chronic pelvic pain, incontinence and obstetric fistula [2].

---

1 Corresponding author: Email: jchamber@mcmaster.ca

Around the world, pregnancy complications kill more 15-19 year-old girls than any other disease or cause [3].

Maternal mortality has beleaguered humankind for thousands of years. It has been written about in historical accounts and immortalized in monuments. The Bible records that Rachel died in childbirth [4] and Emperor Shah Jahan constructed the Taj Mahal in memory of his wife, the Empress Mumtaz Mahal, who died in 1630 from a postpartum hemorrhage at her fourteenth delivery [5].

Much of the world had become inured to the devastating effect of maternal mortality. During the twentieth century, most of the developed world improved primary healthcare for the majority of their citizens and, in doing so, included the provision of maternal healthcare. Since then, the great divide between rates of mothers dying in the developed versus the developing world has widened enormously.

At last, in 1987 at the Safe Motherhood Conference in Nairobi, the world's attention became focused on the tolerated tragedy of maternal deaths in developing countries. Other conferences followed, including the International Conference on Population and Development (ICPD) in Cairo in 1994. The organization for Economic Co-operation and Development (OECD) in 2000 set the International Development Target (IDT) of reducing maternal mortality 75% by 2015 [6]. The Fifth Millennium Development Goal targeted the reduction of maternal mortality by 75% between 1990 and 2015, with the aim of having all deliveries attended by a skilled health provider [7].

At present, there is an attempt to create global public health programs which reduce maternal mortality; however, the challenges have been greater than initially anticipated. Models for successful, globally initiated public health programs exist. A good example is the Global Polio Eradication Plan, which has gone to the people and has been sustained with international cooperation. Consequently, polio is now eradicated in all but six countries worldwide [8].

The success of the polio program is due in part to its mobile and flexible delivery system. In contrast, accessibility for all mothers to safe child bearing requires 24/7 care and stable, appropriate facilities. The debate on how to best deliver such services has been ongoing and opinions differ with respect to the remedy. Program planners have focused on several strategies, including the provision of antenatal care and training of Traditional Birth Attendants (TBA's), as magic bullets for safe motherhood. However, the results of these strategies have been disappointing, as worldwide rates of maternal mortality have barely changed over the past twenty years [9].

THE SCOPE OF THE PROBLEM

Every day, nearly 1500 mothers die from pregnancy complications. That is the equivalent of three jumbo jets, filled with pregnant mothers, crashing daily. The majority of these women live in the Global South or the developing world. The estimated global number of maternal deaths in 2000 was 529,000 [10]. A maternal death is defined as the death of a woman while pregnant or within 42 days of termination of pregnancy, irrespective of the duration and site of pregnancy, from any cause related to or aggravated by the pregnancy or its management but not from accidental or incidental causes [11]. At least 15% of all pregnant mothers will have a life threatening complication [12]. In some parts of the world (eg. Yemen, Uganda), the fertility rate is just over 7 children per woman of reproductive age [13]. Rates of maternal mortality are very high in countries where women deliver so many babies at home, attended by unskilled individuals, with no hope of timely transfer to facilities offering adequate care.

Public health measures have improved in the developing world. However, maternal mortality and morbidity have not reflected this change. It is still one of the health indicators with the largest discrepancy amongst public health statistics between developed and developing nations [14].

WHERE MOTHERS DIE

The discrepancy in the rates of mothers dying among various regions of the world is staggering. In many cases, the difference is several hundred fold. Of all maternal deaths, almost half were in Africa (251,000) and the other in Asia (253,000) with 4% (22,000) in Latin America and the Caribbean and the remaining less than 1% in the developed world [15]. Maternal mortality (MMR) can be expressed by the maternal mortality ratio (number of maternal deaths per 100,000 live births) with the highest ratios being found in Africa (830 maternal deaths/100,000 live births), Asia (330 deaths) and Oceania (240 deaths). The MMR in Latin America and the Caribbean is 190 and while, in developed countries, the MMR is only 20 deaths/100,000 live births [16].

Table 1. Maternal mortality ratio estimates by United Nations Millennium Development Goal Regions 2000.

Region	MMR	Number of maternal deaths	Lifetime risk of maternal death 1 in
WORLD Total	400	529,000	74
Developed regions	20	2,500	2,800
Developing regions	440	527,000	61
Northern Africa	130	4600	210
Sub-Saharan Africa	920	247,000	16
Asia	330	253,000	94
Eastern Asia	55	11,000	840
South central	520	207,000	46
South east	210	25,000	140
Western Asia	190	9,800	120
Latin America and Caribbean	190	22,000	160
Oceania	240	530	83

Used with permission by WHO. Maternal mortality in 2000. Estimates developed by WHO, UNICEF and UNFPA. Geneva 2004.

When Mothers Die

Most maternal deaths (76%) occur during delivery or directly after, especially within 24 hours of delivery [18]. Access to timely and quality emergency obstetrical care is crucial. The average interval from the onset of postpartum bleeding to death is two hours [19].

Why Mothers Die

Worldwide, the most common cause of maternal death is hemorrhage (bleeding), the two major types being bleeding prior to delivery (antepartum hemorrhage) and bleeding after delivery (postpartum hemorrhage). However, a recent systemic review of maternal mortality by the World Health Organization (WHO) determined that there is a wide regional variation in the causes of maternal deaths. For example, while hemorrhage was the leading cause of death in Africa (33.9%) and Asia (30.8%), hypertensive disorders were the most common cause in Latin America and the Caribbean (25.7%) [20]. In the developed world (for example Canada) hemorrhage is not the leading direct cause of maternal mortality, but rather it is pulmonary embolism and hypertension [21]. Pulmonary embolism is a condition that is much more difficult to diagnose and treat. The preventable causes of death have been adequately dealt with in the majority of the developed world.

Previously, the most commonly cited study of the causes of maternal mortality showed the global distribution of maternal deaths to be hemorrhage (25%), indirect causes (20%), infection (15%), abortion (13%), eclampsia and hypertension (12%), obstructed labour (8%), and indirect causes (8%) [22]. This WHO study helped to quantify the differences in causes of maternal mortality in various regions, illustrating that the causes are not uniform.

Another cause of maternal mortality is abortion. The rates of death due to abortion, according to the WHO study, were highest in Latin America and the Caribbean (12.0%) and lower in Asia (5.7%) and Africa (3.9%) [23]. However, there were wide variations in rates between studies within the various regions and underreporting in some countries, probably skewing the final figures [24]. In the developed world, where safe abortions are usually more accessible, the contribution to maternal deaths by abortions was 8.2% [25]. Regardless of geography or political environment, abortion contributes significantly to maternal deaths.

Another important factor in maternal mortality and morbidity is HIV/AIDS. In 2005, 17.3 million women worldwide were infected with HIV/AIDS with the greatest number being in sub-Saharan Africa. In South Africa, one in four pregnant women was HIV positive [26]. Other treatable diseases such as malaria significantly contribute to maternal and neonatal mortality. Malaria predisposes mothers to anemia and subsequently increases their risk of hemorrhage and death [27].

If Mothers Survive

It is estimated that 300 million women suffer today from pregnancy-related complications including anaemia, uterine prolapse, fistulae (hole in the bladder or rectum that leads to leakage of fluids into vagina), pelvic inflammatory disease and infertility [28]. Many women suffer from a lifelong disability due to these complications of pregnancy. Women with fistulas are profoundly affected by their lack of maternal healthcare—they are incontinent of urine or feces and become social outcasts who are usually infertile and rejected by their husbands and sometimes even by their extended family. Specialized fistula hospitals have been established to repair the physical damage these women have suffered, but the psychological and social problems can sometimes be a greater barrier.

Women who are at highest risk of dying from pregnancy complications are at the extreme of ages—either the very young or very old [29]. In the developing world, many young girls are married before their bodies and pelvic structures have had a chance to fully mature. This leads to young girls bearing babies and their birth canal is not large enough for the fetus to pass through. Instead, the fetus remains in the birth canal for days while the young girl labours in pain and without any relief. Often the fetus will die and finally be passed out, leaving the young mother with a torn and damaged birth canal. She soon notices urine and stool passing spontaneously from the vagina. She has developed an obstetrical fistula—a condition that will leave her permanently impaired and as a social outcast unless she is fortunate enough to obtain a rare successful operation.

Mothers who have delivered many children are also at higher risk of dying in subsequent pregnancies [30]. Women who have delivered five or more children (known as grand multiparous) face higher risks of bleeding after delivery and dying from high blood pressure [31].

THE EFFECTS OF MATERNAL MORTALITY: IF A MOTHER DIES

A) Lost Children

If a mother dies, the entire family is affected by the loss of this important family member. In fact, if a mother dies leaving behind infants and children less than five years of age, those remaining children are more likely to die [32]. Those who survive are often given away to other family members who have large families with the result that these small children do not experience the careful attention of their natural mother. They fall victim to preventable diseases that could have been treated early or totally prevented through immunizations. The fetus/newborn that the deceased mother delivers is also at a very high risk of dying. The newborn has no source of natural nourishment and must be usually fed with formula— another source of potential infection for the newborn.

Each year, 3.3 million babies are stillborn and another four million die within 28 days of birth. Ninety eight (98%) percent of these deaths are in the developing world. The main causes of these neonatal/stillborn deaths are intrinsically linked to poor maternal health or death. In other words, when the mother is poorly cared for, not only one but two people may die or become permanently disabled [33]. It is estimated that improved maternal health could reduce newborn death rates by 40% [34].

In addition to the orphans caused by poor maternal healthcare, the death toll from HIV/AIDS has currently left 15.2 million children living as orphans, while 2.3 million children actually have the disease, primarily caused by mother to child transmission [35].

B) Lost Potential

Mothers are responsible in the developing world for the care and nurture of children but their contribution to the economy itself is significant. When a mother dies in childbirth, there is a significant loss, not only to the immediate family but also the larger economy in general. The REDUCE model estimates the cost of maternal/neonatal ill health using a human capital approach and productivity losses. It estimates that in Uganda alone, 84.86 Million US$ is lost each year due to poor maternal and newborn health [36].

In an attempt to measure the overall burden of disease due to losses from premature death and non fatal disability, the 'Disability Adjusted Life Year' (DALY) was created. It is a time-based indicator of health outcomes [37]. DALY's can be used to evaluate the cost-effectiveness of maternity health services or interventions; however they can underestimate the true burden of maternal mortality in addition to undervaluing the cost-effectiveness of an intervention [38].

WHAT ARE THE BARRIERS?

A) Is it Money?

Most maternal deaths occur in poor countries. However, the link to poor maternal health and low resources is not a simple relationship. There are significant differences in maternal mortality ratios between countries with similar Gross Domestic Products (GDP) [39].

B) Is it the Training and Use of Traditional Birth Attendants (TBA's)?

Traditional birth attendants can be found in most communities although their roles and appearance are very different. The WHO defines a TBA to be a 'person who assists the mother during childbirth and who initially acquired her skills by delivering babies herself or by working with others' [40]. Traditional birth attendants are usually illiterate older women who will take payment in kind for their services often rendered in the home of the traditional birth attendant herself [41]. This is in contrast to the skilled midwife who usually only works in health facilities where cash payments only are accepted. Some TBA's deliver as few as two to three babies per year while others delivery up to twenty [42].

The debate continues to rage about the role of TBA training in the developing world. One major problem is the lack of accurate and well planned evaluation of the training programs. Some studies report that TBA's do practice what they learn [42] however extra confidence can also backfire as it may lead to an increase in dangerous practices with subsequent delay in referral [44]. The stumbling block seems to be the effective treatment of pregnancy complications. China reduced its maternal mortality ratio from 1500 to 115 maternal deaths per 100,000 live births [45] by providing maternity services with minimally trained village birth attendants but having a strong back up referral network. On the other hand, Malaysia, Sri Lanka and Thailand have all reduced maternal mortality ratios by gradually instituting coverage of Emergency Obstetrical Care (EOC) with professional attendants [46]. In contrast, the maternal mortality ratio in Bangladesh has remained static despite many years of TBA training and continual lack of EOC [47]. Research has shown that the training of TBA's has not contributed to the reduction of maternal mortality since it tends to cause governments to view the importance of access of skilled attendants for all mothers with much less urgency [48].

Trained TBA's are more likely to practice hygienic deliveries than untrained TBA's however, there is no difference in postpartum infections [49]. An entire book could be written on the challenges and proposed benefits of TBA training. In the absence of a strong referral system and support to hospital services to provide EOC, there is no conclusive evidence that TBA training alone can prevent maternal death [50]. The need to effectively transition from untrained TBA's to competent caring professional attendants is a difficult yet essential progression. The challenge remains in the middle ground as countries plan how to make this goal a reality while gleaning the potential benefits of the significant role and place that TBA's currently have in many communities.

C) Is it Antenatal Care?

There is little evidence to support that antenatal care can reduce maternal mortality in and of itself [51]. It must be part of a system of care that provides Emergency Obstetrical Care (EOC) with competent staff [53]. The World Health Organization has recommended four visits for low risk pregnant women based on a large trial [53]. In 1978, the WHO had developed the 'risk approach' concept for pregnant women [54]. The approach tried to identify risk factors so that the care could be delivered to individuals in need. A high false positive, false negative rate proved the approach not to be successful on a larger scale. Instead, every pregnant woman is now viewed to be at risk and therefore a system where all women can access Emergency Obstetrical Care is essential [55].

D) Is it Measurement?

Measuring maternal mortality is difficult for several reasons. Three pieces of information must be known -- the number of deaths of women of reproductive age, pregnancy status and medical causes of death. This information must be acquired in settings where there is no vital statistics registry of deaths (especially for women of reproductive age), no medical certificates of death and pregnancy status is withheld, especially in early gestations, which are thought to be a private matter. Under-reporting and misclassifications are very real and significant problems [56]. Approaches to obtaining data on the levels of maternal mortality include: 1) ensuring the use of the vital statistics registration; 2) direct household survey methods; 3) indirect or direct sisterhood methods; 4) reproductive age mortality studies (RAMOS) 5) verbal autopsy, and 6) census. Each approach has its strengths and weaknesses along with varying degrees of accuracy [57].

Since measuring maternal mortality is difficult, it is equally challenging to measure the impact of interventions aimed at reducing maternal mortality and morbidity. More recently, there have been a large number of health indicators that have been developed and tested. Indicators vary based on the situation and the geographical area being covered. In 1996, the

World Health Organization held an interagency meeting which led to 15 global indicators for monitoring progress of reproductive health targets at a national and global level. Two more indicators were subsequently added which targeted HIV/AIDS [58]. These reproductive health indicators include total fertility rate, contraceptive prevalence, maternal mortality ratio, percentage of women attended at least once during pregnancy by skilled health personnel, percentage of births attended by skilled health personnel and number of facilities with basic and comprehensive essential obstetric care per 500,000 population. All health indicators are subject to limitations caused by lack of routine data collection and inadequate measurement techniques. The challenge in measuring effective interventions continues. See Table 2 for list of health indicators and definitions.

Table 2. Partial list of reproductive health indicators for global monitoring.

Total fertility rate—Total number of children a woman would have by the end of her reproductive period if she experienced the currently prevailing age-specific fertility rates throughout her child bearing life

Contraceptive prevalence—Percentage of women of reproductive age (15-49) who are using (or whose partner is using) a contraceptive method at a particular point in time

Maternal mortality ratio—the number of maternal deaths per 100 000 live births

Percentage of women attended at least once during pregnancy by skilled health personnel for reasons relating to pregnancy—percentage of women attended at least once during pregnancy, by skilled health personnel (excluding trained or untrained traditional birth attendants) for reasons relating to pregnancy

Percentage of births attended by skilled health personnel—Percentage of births attended by skilled health personnel (excluding trained and untrained traditional birth attendants)

Taken from Measuring Access to Reproductive Health Services. Report of WHO/UNFPA Technical Consultation 2-3 December 2003 Annex 2: Seventeen reproductive health indicators short-listed for global monitoring pg 11.

E) Is it Cultural?

The physical causes or diagnoses of maternal mortality have been reported in depth in the WHO study [59]. The majority of these causes can be treated or prevented. However, the larger picture of why mothers don't receive these treatments in a timely fashion continues to impede international efforts to improve maternal health. The contributing causes that lead to maternal death were initially described as the three delays of maternal mortality [60]. The first delay is in the decision to seek care. Many times women have to wait for their husband's permission in order to seek care or the woman herself may not recognize that she has a complication that requires treatment. The 'wait and see' tendency leads to mothers presenting late for care. The second delay is transport. Many regions have no accessible roads or means of transport. Other women require financial resources in order to access the available transportation but she has no money. The third delay is at the level of the health care facility. Medical staff or life saving medication may not be available to treat her maternal complication.

The slogan 'Every Pregnancy Faces Risk' was made popular by the World Health Organization. The statement helps to bring out the association between the high maternal mortality ratios (MMR) in countries/regions with high total fertility rates. In Sub-Saharan Africa, the total fertility rate is 5.6 children per woman of reproductive age while the MMR is 920 maternal deaths per 100,000 live births. To contrast, in North America, the total fertility rate is 2 children per woman while the MMR is only 16 maternal deaths per 100,000 live births [61].

In general, the positive association between high fertility and high maternal mortality rates holds true. Addressing high fertility rates is a crucial step in reducing maternal mortality in the developing world. Major barriers such as poverty and illiteracy along with the desire for large family sizes, all contribute to high fertility rates and a low use of family planning methods [62]. Women can feel that unless they are producing a large number of children, they are not contributing to the family well being and may be replaced. Dispelling family planning myths and educating individuals and communities about child spacing in addition to ensuring an adequate and reliable source of family planning methods, are key strategies in decreasing fertility rates and subsequently reducing maternal mortality and morbidity [63].

E) Is it a Lack of Human Rights?

The discussion about maternal mortality and morbidity cannot be complete without reviewing the interaction between these tragedies and the issue of human rights, specifically reproductive rights. Women's capacity to exercise their reproductive rights has benefits for their own personal well being and health as well as that of their family and community. Mothers are less likely to die during pregnancy, their infants are more likely to survive into childhood and their girl children are more likely to complete primary and secondary education. Women are more able to protect themselves from sexually transmitted infections and they become more actively involved in decision making both for their own lives and that of the community [64].

These are substantial outcomes that are intrinsically linked to a woman's ability to exercise her reproductive rights—rights that have been agreed on by governments worldwide. Reproductive rights are sometimes confused by some to be equated only with the right to terminate a pregnancy, which is an incorrect assumption. Reproductive rights can be grouped into the following clusters: 1) the right to life, survival, security and sexuality; 2) the right to self-determination and free choice of maternity; 3) health and the benefits of scientific progress; 4) non-discrimination and due respect for difference; and 5) information, education and decision-making [65].

When a mother dies due to pregnancy complications, her country of residence has failed in its obligation to guarantee a dignified existence (rights cluster one). A young woman who has undergone female genital cutting has been denied the right to liberty and security of person. She also has a higher chance of dying from pregnancy complications. Young girls who are married off at 12 years of age are denied the right to choose to marry and to have children (rights cluster two). These girls are more likely to succumb to pregnancy complications. The 'special protection accorded to mothers during a reasonable period before and after childbirth' which is mandated in the Economic Covenant (Article 10 (2)) is a basic reproductive right that is a distant reality for millions of women around the world [66].

The right to basic health, guaranteed by the majority of the world's states in the Universal Declaration of Human Rights nearly six decades ago, (1948) [67], is still far from a reality for most pregnant mothers around the world. A myriad of other treaties and conventions have called for the same basic right to health but the actual implementation of these agreements into national policies and health care delivery, remain a major barrier to health for the majority of women in the developing world. The lack of human rights for millions of women are around the world cannot be more apparent than when one examines the dearth of health services and grim statistics for a millions of mothers in the developing world.

INITIATING CHANGE: THE CHALLENGES

Why Change is Challenging

With so many partners committed to the cause of improving maternal health, it is often difficult to reconcile the slow rate in the improvement of maternal health. Often, the problem of poor coordination of plans can be an obstacle and few organizations focus primarily on maternal health. The health of mothers is one of many pressing needs. At times, there has been a disjoint between the need to improve maternal health facilities and personnel and the need for the society itself to be mobilized. Various models of social mobilization have been created including policy advocacy, community mobilization, social marketing and behavior change communication. Clearly, individual behavioral change and an enabling environment are needed. Shared responsibility amongst all stakeholders including individuals, organizations, health care providers and policy makers is essential to make safe motherhood as a shared responsibility for all [68].

Social mobilization requires a trans-disciplinary approach to health. All sectors are needed to be involved in promoting and maximizing maternal health. A new innovative program in Uganda is strategically training leaders from various professions and expertise to be champions for maternal health within their own profession. The program is called 'Save the Mothers' [69]. The leaders being trained under the program must complete a project within their own sphere of expertise/experience prior to their graduation with a masters in public health leadership. The program is building a network of dedicated individuals including leaders within the field of politics, journalism, faith communities, education, law and social sciences.

In the early days of maternal child health programs (MCH), there was a focus on child health at the expense of the mother ("Where's the M in MCH?"). However, many planners are now sensitive to the special focus that maternal health requires in order to facilitate real change.[70]

THE FIRST CHALLENGE – FOCUS

The first challenge in attaining safe motherhood was to make the issue as a focus for international concern and action. Safe motherhood became a recognized part of the definition of reproductive health in the Programme of Action in 1994 at the International Conference on Population and Development. Several large meetings and conferences have been held with the focus of developing international strategies that will work to reduce maternal mortality. The goals have been lofty and their implementation has been challenging.

The Safe Motherhood Technical Consultation in Sri Lanka 1997 identified 10 action agendas that were thought to be important foundations in the advancement of safe motherhood. These include: 1) advance safe motherhood through human rights, 2) empowering women and their choices and 3) presenting safe motherhood as a vital social and economic investment. Other action messages include 4) delay marriage and first birth, 5) recognizing that all pregnancies face risk (and not just those with a high antenatal screen), 6) advocating skilled attendants for all deliveries and 7) improving the access of quality maternal health services for all women. The group also called for 8) increased access to family planning to avoid unplanned pregnancy and address unsafe abortion. Organizations were called upon to build partnerships that advocate for safe motherhood and to make the effort to measure the progress of these particular interventions [71].

THE SECOND CHALLENGE – IMPROVED CARE

Individuals and communities must be encouraged to understand that a safe pregnancy and delivery do not merely happen by chance. In order to realize improvement in maternal health, skilled birth attendants (whether in facilities or communities) should be the backbone of maternal health services according to the Millennium Development Goals Task Force on Child and Maternal Health. A skilled attendant refers exclusively to people with midwifery skills (for example, doctors, midwives and nurses) who have been trained to proficiency in the skills necessary to manage normal deliveries and diagnose, manage or refer complications [72]. These attendants should be integrated into a health system that will support, supervise and supply the functioning needs of these skilled attendants [73].

Improved antenatal care can create important opportunities to discuss birth preparedness with a pregnant woman and others who may accompany her. She should be encouraged to make a birth plan with her provider, partner and family. In addition, she should be able to recognize danger signs and know the transportation system and where to go in case of emergency [74]. See Table 3 for a list of effective antenatal interventions.

An important development in the coordination of these groups is the formation of International alliances such as the White Ribbon Alliance (WRA). This coalition is broad and helps to expand the agenda of safe motherhood by creating a collective identity around an issue. The strength of this coalition is that it is not dependent on one single NGO but works to unify various organizations even when some of their basic definitions may be different. Another group, the Maternal and Neonatal Health Program (MNH) focused its program on birth preparedness and complication readiness [75].

The need to integrate safe motherhood services and practices with HIV prevention, testing and treatment has never been greater. The challenge is to ensure that both are equally and effectively promoted as basic human rights.

Table 3. A modified list of antenatal interventions known to be effective.

Condition	Test or treatment
1. prevention of anemia	routine iron and folate during pregnancy
	Malaria chemoprophylaxis
2. detection, investigation of anemia	copper sulphate test
	colorimetric tests
	Packed cell volume
	Coulter counter
3. treatment of iron deficiency anemia	oral iron
	I.M. or I.V. iron
	packed cell transfusion
4. detection, investigation of pregnancy induced hypertension	blood pressure
	testing clean urine
5. treatment of severe preeclampsia	transfer for expert care
6. screening for infection	serology for syphilis
	Microbiology for gonnorhoea
	Bacteruria screening
7. primary prevention of Infection	tetanus immunization in pregnancy or
	women of child bearing age

Adapted from Antenatal interventions known to be effective (adapted from Rooney 1992) in Safe Motherhood Strategies: A Review of the Evidence ed by V De Brouwere and W Van Lerberghe, Studies in Health Services Organization and Policy (17), 2001 p 41 . Used with permission.

THE THIRD CHALLENGE: FINANCIAL PRIORITY

Maternal health must become a national priority that is backed by financial support and human resources. Both local governments and international aid organizations need to increase funding so that health systems, particularly at the district level, are accessible to the poorest mother [76]. Skilled attendants are a priority within the system yet many developing countries are being ravaged by a mass exodus of skilled workers to greener pastures abroad. Strategies are needed to both train and retain these important life saving attendants [77].

THE FOURTH CHALLENGE: EVIDENCE BASED PRACTICE STANDARDS

On a national level, attempts to improve access and quality of obstetric care have been made through the use of 'Confidential Enquiries in Maternal Deaths' [78]. Evidence based practice guidelines have been developed based on scientific literature [79] and can be used to establish criteria of best practice in obstetric care. These external criteria can be negotiated as internal standards for the audit group who must also take into consideration the local circumstances or limitations [80].

MAKING A DIFFERENCE

Recognizing the differences in the causes of maternal mortality in various regions is an important undertaking in order to guide policy planning and programming in the reduction of maternal mortality. Regional and global conferences such as the Post Partum Hemorrhage (PPH) Initiative in Uganda (Apr 5-8, 2006) (sponsored by USAID) are important in building consensus and cooperation in the treatment of maternal mortality especially in initiating new methods in the treatment of postpartum hemorrhage (eg. misoprostol for PPH) and encouraging the abandonment of those less helpful (eg. ergometrine as a first line drug for PPH) [81]. The treatment of hypertension in pregnancy and eclampsia are also well known especially the importance of stocking magnesium sulphate (the treatment and prevention of eclampsia) in all maternal units and particularly in Latin America/Caribbean. In all regions, the planning of pregnancies is a vital strategy to reducing the role of abortion in mothers dying [82]. Accessible, affordable and acceptable means of family planning are essential to prevent the tragedy of lives lost due to abortion.

Most mothers' die within 24 hours of delivery. This is an important fact to focus on as one develops strategies to reduce maternal mortality. The most important time to prevent maternal death is right around the time of delivery. Interventions around the time of delivery will have a great impact on maternal mortality.

Access to skilled attendance at birth has been a strategy that has successfully reduced maternal mortality [83]. Several developing countries have combined quality primary health care with referral care as a focused strategy. This has led to maternal mortality ratios dropping in considerably short time frames. Table Four shows the developing countries who increased midwifery care and access to hospital referral—their rates fell dramatically.

Table 4. Number of years to halve maternal mortality in selected countries.

	From 400 to 200	From 200 to 100	From 100 to 50
In 11-12 years	Thailand '62-'74		
In 9-10 years	Sri Lanka '56-'65	Honduras '68-'78 Malaysia '65-'75	
In 7-8 years		Sri Lanka '66-74 Thailand '74-81	Malaysia '75-83
In 4-6 years		Chili '71-'77	Thailand '81-'85

Taken from Safe Motherhood Strategies: A Review of the Evidence ed by V De Brouwere and W Van Lerberghe, Studies in Health Services Organization and Policy (17), 2001 p 2 . Used with permission.

At the same time, simply increasing access to midwifery care and hospital based referrals is not enough to meet the demands of mothers in the developing world. The need for quality of care and sensitivity to mothers' needs cannot be overlooked [84]. When mothers are treated with substandard care, their privacy neglected and their wishes for a particular birth position are ridiculed, many choose to stay home and risk the consequences.

Professionals, both at the primary health care level and at the hospital institutions need to be responsible and accountable [85]. Few tools are available to effectively measure these factors although quality assurance programs may contribute [86]. In the long run, both peer pressure and client demand will have to ensure the accountability and responsibility that are already expected in many developed countries [87].

The plight of mothers dying from pregnancy complications and suffering significant illness as a result of untreated complications has begun to attract international attention. Numerous international organizations, non-governmental organizations (NGO's) and national health ministries have attempted to confront the tragedy through various methods and means of approaches. Some have been more successful than others.

The United Nations' arm called the United Nations Fund for Population (UNFPA) is focused primarily on reproductive health issues and particularly on the health of women. The United National International Children's Emergency Fund (UNICEF) has also recognized the important roles of mothers in the lives of children's health and are addressing the need to improve the health of those who primarily care for children. The World Health Organization (WHO) has developed several strategies including the program 'Making Pregnancy Safer' in order to enhance maternal health through various public campaigns and the development of important training manuals which are essential for standard setting in maternal health care settings.

In 1987, the global Safe Motherhood Initiative was launched in Nairobi, Kenya. It was sponsored by several United Nations agencies including the United Nations Children's Emergency Fund (UNICEF), United Nations Population Fund (UNFPA), the World Bank, the World Health Organization (WHO), International Planned Parenthood (IPPF) and the Population Council. Together, the group formed the Safe Motherhood Inter-Agency Group (IAG). Professional organizations such as the International Confederation of Midwives and the Federation of International Obstetricians and Gynecologist have since joined the coalition. In many circumstances, the international agencies merge their resources and expertise in order to deliver a better product [88].

External government sponsored programs from the U.S., Britain, Sweden, Canada, Norway and others (ie. USAID, DFID, SIDA, CIDA) target maternal health. USAID sponsors some agencies which are targeting maternal health (eg. CARE, EngenderHealth, Access, JHPIEGO, Save the Children and others). Other NGO's include the White Ribbon Alliance, the Regional Prevention of Maternal Mortality (Africa), the Averting Maternal Death and Disability Program (supported by the Gates Foundation through the Millman's School of Public Health, Columbia University) and IMMPACT (Initiative for Maternal Mortality Program Assessment through the University of Aberdeen UK) along with a host of others.

Professional organizations such as the Federation of International Obstetricians/ Gynecologists (FIGO) and the International Federation of Midwives (IFM) are also promoting the sharing of expertise and knowledge in the care of pregnant women. Partnerships have been developed between professional obstetrical associations between developed and developing countries [89]. These kinds of activities help not only to improve the situation for mothers in those countries but also to raise the profile and importance of safe maternal health.

CONCLUSION

As the timelines of the Millennium Development Goals approach, particularly those relating to maternal health, it is evident that the attainment of these goals may still be a distant dream. High maternal mortality and morbidity rates, low use of skilled attendants and even lower utilization of modern contraceptive methods, continue to be major challenges for communities, governments and international organizations to address. The promotion of women's rights and education play an important role in realizing sustainable and real improvement. A trans-disciplinary approach to safe motherhood is essential to effectively tackle the major causes of maternal mortality and morbidity. The causes and treatments of life threatening complications have been known for years but the capacity to bring the cure to the needy mothers of the world has proved to be a much bigger challenge.

REFERENCES

[1]   *Maternal Mortality in 2000*: Estimates developed by WHO, UNICEF, UNFPA. 2004. World Health Organization, Geneva, pg 1

[2]   UNFPA, *Mortality Update 2002* (UNFPA, New York, 2003)

[3]   UNICEF, *Innocent Digest: Early Marriage 7*, New York, UNICEF, Mar 2001

[4]   *The Holy Bible Genesis* 35:17-18

[5]   Reference from *www.taj-mahal-india.travel.com*

[6]   Organisation for Economic Co-operation and Development (OECD) 2000. *A Better World for All: Progress towards the International Development Goals*. OECD, Paris.

[7]   World Health Report 2003 *Shaping the Future* www.who.int/whr pg 28

[8]   *Global Polio Erradication Initiative Strategic Plan 2004-2008*. WHO, UNICEF, CDC. WHO, Geneva 2003

[9]   Van Lerberghe W, De Brouwere V. Reducing maternal mortality in a context of poverty. *In Safe Motherhood Strategies: A Review of the Evidence*. ITG Press, Belgium. Studies in Health Services Organization and Policy, 17, 2001 p 1

[10]   *Maternal Mortality in 2000*. Estimates developed by WHO, UNICEF and UNFPA. WHO, Geneva, 2004. p 1

[11]   WHO, *International Statistical Classification of Diseases and Related Health Problems. Tenth Revision*, Geneva, WHO, 1992

[12]   *Guidelines for Monitoring Availability and Use of Obstetric Services*. UNICEF, WHO, UNFPA. UNICEF, New York, 1997, pg 1 www.unicef.org

[13]   Progress Since the World Summit for Children—a Statistical Review. Summarized in *Monitoring the Situation of Women and Children*, UNICEF, www.childinfo.org

[14]   *State of the World's Population 2004*. The Cairo Consensus at Ten: Population, Reproductive Health and the Global Effort to End Poverty. UNFPA, New York, 2004

[15]   *Maternal Mortality in 2000*. Estimates developed by WHO, UNICEF and UNFPA. WHO, Geneva, 2004. p 1

[16]   *Maternal Mortality in 2000*. Estimates developed by WHO, UNICEF and UNFPA. WHO, Geneva, 2004. p 2

[17] *Maternal Mortality in 2000.* Estimates developed by WHO, UNICEF and UNFPA. WHO, Geneva, 2004. p 2

[18] Safe Motherhood Action Agenda: Priorities for the next decade. Report on Safe Motherhood Technical Consultation 13-23 October 1997, Colombo Sri Lanka. *Family Care International.* Prepared by Ann Starrs. p 37

[19] Safe Motherhood Action Agenda: Priorities for the next decade. Report on Safe Motherhood Technical Consultation 13-23 October 1997, Colombo Sri Lanka. *Family Care International.* Prepared by Ann Starrs. p 39.

[20] Khan K, Wojdyla D, Say L, Gulmezoglu M, Van Look P. WHO Analysis of causes of maternal death: a systematic review. *The Lancet 2006*, 367:1066-1074

[21] *Special Report on Maternal Mortality and Severe Morbidity in Canada. Enhanced Surveillance.* Ed by Rusen ID, Liston R, published by Public Health Agency of Canada *http://www.phac-aspc.gc.ca*

[22] AbouZahr C, Royston E. *Maternal mortality: a global factbook.* WHO/MCH/MSM 91.3. Geneva: World Health Organization, 1991

[23] Khan K, Wojdyla D, Say L, Gulmezoglu M, Van Look P. WHO Analysis of causes of maternal death: a systematic review. *The Lancet 2006*, 367:1066-1074

[24] Khan K, Wojdyla D, Say L, Gulmezoglu M, Van Look P. WHO Analysis of causes of maternal death: a systematic review. *The Lancet 2006*, 367:1066-1074

[25] Khan K, Wojdyla D, Say L, Gulmezoglu M, Van Look P. WHO Analysis of causes of maternal death: a systematic review. *The Lancet 2006*, 367:1066-1074

[26] 2006 Report on the global AIDS epidemic, *UNAIDS*, May 2006. *www.unaids.org/en/HIV_data/2006Global Report*

[27] *Reducing Maternal Deaths: The Challenge of the New Millennium in the African Region.* WHO—Regional Office for Africa, Republic of Congo *www.afro.who.int/drh*

[28] Safe Motherhood Action Agenda: Priorities for the next decade. Report on Safe Motherhood Technical Consultation 13-23 October 1997, Colombo Sri Lanka. *Family Care International.* Prepared by Ann Starrs. p 1

[29] WHO Fact Sheet "Making Pregnancy Safer" *Fact sheet #26*, Feb 2004

[30] Every Pregnancy Faces Risk. *World Health Day. Safe Motherhood* (WHO 98.5) WHO Reproductive health, Geneva 7 Apr 1998

[31] *Antenatal Care: Report of a technical working group, 1996.* World Health Organization, 1996 www.who.int/reproductive-health/publications

[32] Katz J, West KP, Khatry SK, Christian P, LeClerg SC, Pradham EK. Risk Factors to early infant mortality in Sarlahi district, Nepal. *WHO Bulleting 2003*, 81: 717-725

[33] *World Health Report 2005: Make Every Mother and Child Count.* World Health Organization, Geneva. Chapter 5

[34] Lawn J, Cousens S, Zupan J. 4 Million neonatal deaths: When, Where, Why? The *Lancet Mar 2005* (365) Issue 9462 p 891-900

[35] 2006 Report on the global AIDS epidemic, *UNAIDS*, May 2006. *www.unaids.org/en/HIV_data/2006Global Report.*

[36] Burkhalter BR. *Assumptions and estimates for the application of REDUCE Safe Motherhood model in Uganda.* Bethesda, MD. Centre for Human Sciences 2001.

[37] *DALYs and Reproductive Health: Report of an informal consultation 27-28 April 1998,* WHO Reproductive Health. 1999 p 4

[38]   Josephine Borghi, What is the cost of maternal health care and how is it financed? In Safe Motherhood Strategies: a Review of the Evidence. Ed Vincent De Brouwere and Wim Van Lerberghe. *Studies in Health Services Organization and Policy*, 16, 2001, ITG Press, Belgium, 2001 p 247

[39]   Van Lerberghet W, de Brouwere V. Reducing maternal mortality in a context of poverty, in In Safe Motherhood Strategies: a Review of the Evidence. Ed Vincent De Brouwere and Wim Van Lerberghe. *Studies in Health Services Organization and Policy,* 16, 2001, ITG Press, Belgium, 2001 p2

[40]   Leedam, E Traditional Birth Attendants. Int. J. Gynaecol. *Obstet 1985* 23,249-274.

[41]   United Nations Population Fund. Support to Traditional Birth Attendants. *Evaluation Findings Issue 7.* December 1996.

[42]   World Health Organization (1997) *Coverage of maternity care: a listing of available information.* WHO, Geneva

[43]   Akpala CO. An evaluation of knowledge and practices of trained traditional birth attendants in Bodinga, Sokoto State, Nigeria. *Journal of Tropical Medicine and Hygiene* (1994) 97, 46-50

[44]   Eades CA, Brace C, Osei L, LaGuardia KD. Traditional birth attendants and maternal mortality in Ghana. *Social Science and Medicine* (1993) 35, 1503-7

[45]   Koblinksy MA, Campbell O and Heichelheim Organizing deliver care: what works for safe motherhood? *Bulletin of the World Health Organization* J (1999): 77(5) 399-406

[46]   Starrs A. The Safe Motherhood Action Agenda: Priorities for the Next Decade. Report on the Safe Motherhood Technical Consultation, 18-23 October, 1997, Colombo, Sri Lanka. New York: *Family Care International* and the Inter-Agency Group for Safe Motherhood

[47]   Nessa S. Training of traditional birth attendants: success and failures in Bangladesh. Int. J. Gynecol. *Obstet.* (1995) 50 (suppl) S135-S139

[48]   Skilled Professional Care at Birth and Afterwards. *World Health Report, Chapter 5,* WHO, Geneva

[49]   Goodburn EA, Chowdhury M, Gazi R, Marshall T and Graham W. Training traditional birth attendants in clean delivery does not prevent postpartum infection. *Health Policy and Planning 2000* 15 (4), 394-399

[50]   Bergstrom S and Goodburn E. The role of traditional birth attendants in the reduction of maternal mortality in Safe Motherhood Strategies: a review of the Evidence. Ed Vincent De Brouwere and Wim Van Lerberghe. *Studies in Health Services Organization and Policy*, 16, 2001, ITG Press, Belgium, 2001 p 89.

[51]   Bergsjo P What is the evidence for the role of antenatal care strategies in the reduction of maternal mortality and morbidity? In Safe Motherhood Strategies: a Review of the Evidence. Ed Vincent De Brouwere and Wim Van Lerberghe. *Studies in Health Services Organization and Policy*, 16, 2001, ITG Press, Belgium, 2001 p 35

[52]   McDonagh M. Is antenatal care effective in reducing maternal morbidity and mortality? *Health Policy and Planning* 1996 11, 1-15

[53]   Villar J, Ba'aqueel G et al. WHO randomized controlled trial for the evaluation of a new model of antenatal care *The Lancet* vol 357 Issue 9268 p 1551-1564

[54]   World Health Organization (1978) Risk Approach for Maternal and Child Health Care. *WHO Offset Publication No. 39.* WHO, Geneva

[55] Bergsjo P What is the evidence for the role of antenatal care strategies in the reduction of maternal mortality and morbidity? In Safe Motherhood Strategies: a Review of the Evidence. Ed Vincent De Brouwere and Wim Van Lerberghe. *Studies in Health Services Organization and Policy*, 16, 2001, ITG Press, Belgium, 2001 p 38

[56] *Maternal Mortality in 2000*. Estimates developed by WHO, UNICEF and UNFPA. WHO, Geneva, 2004. p 4

[57] *Maternal Mortality in 2000*. Estimates developed by WHO, UNICEF and UNFPA. WHO, Geneva, 2004 p 5

[58] World Health Organization. Measuring Access to Reproductive Health Services. *Report of WHO/UNFPA Technical Consultation 2-3* December 2003. WHO, Geneva 2005.

[59] Khan K, Wojdyla D, Say L, Gulmezoglu M, Van Look P. WHO Analysis of causes of maternal death: a systematic review. *The Lancet* 2006, 367:1066-1074

[60] Thaddeus S, Maine D. Too Far to Walk: Maternal Mortality in Context. *Social Science and Medicine*. 1994, 38:1091-1110

[61] Women of Our World. *Population Reference Bureau*. 2005 *www.prb.org/2000women*

[62] *World Development Indicators*, World Bank 2006, Washington Chapter 2 People *http://devdata.worldbank.org/wdi2006/*

[63] Safe Motherhood Action Agenda: Priorities for the Next Decade; report on Safe Motherhood Technical Consultation October 18-3, 1997 Colombo Sri Lanka. 1997, *Family Care International*

[64] Public Choices, Private Decisions: Sexual and Reproductive Health and the Millennium Development Goals. *UN Millennium Project Report* by Stan Bernstein and Charlotte Juul Hansen 2006 *http://www.unmillenniumproject.org/.*

[65] Cook R, Dickens B, Fathalla, M. *Reproductive Health and Human Rights*. Oxford 2003 p 158-185

[66] Cook R, Dickens B, Fathalla, M. *Reproductive Health and Human Rights*. Oxford 2003 p 158-185

[67] *Declaration of Human Rights* December 8, 1948. See *www.ohchr.org* for full text

[68] Igniting Change! Accelerating Collective Action for Reproductive Health and Safe Motherhood. *Joint thematic paper of ENABLE project and the Maternal and Neonatal Health Program* by Nancy Russell and Mart Levitt-Dayal. Aug 2003 Bureau for Global Health, p 6-7

[69] see *www.savethemothers.org*

[70] Rosenfield A, Maine D. Maternal mortality—a neglected tragedy. Where is the 'M' in MCH? *Lancet* July 1985 13:2 (8446) 83-5. .

[71] Safe Motherhood Action Agenda: Priorities for the Next Decade; report on Safe Motherhood Technical Consultation October 18-3, 1997 Colombo Sri Lanka. 1997, *Family Care International*

[72] *Reduction of Maternal Mortality: a joint statement.* WHO/UNFPA/ UNICEF/ World Bank. Geneva, WHO, 1999

[73] 'Who's Got the Power: Transforming Health Systems for Women and Children, *UN Millennium Project*, 2006 printed by Earthscan and UN publications http://www.unmillenniumproject.org/documents/maternalchild-complete.pdf

[74] Birth Preparedness and Complication Readiness: A matrix of shared responsibility. Maternal and Neonatal Health Program, Baltimore 2004

[75] Igniting Change! Accelerating Collective Action for Reproductive Health and Safe Motherhood. *Joint thematic paper of ENABLE project and the Maternal and Neonatal Health Program* by Nancy Russell and Mart Levitt-Dayal. Aug 2003 Bureau for Global Health, p 7

[76] Who's Got the Power: Transforming Health Systems for Women and Children, *UN Millennium Project*, 2006 printed by Earthscan and UN publications *http://www.unmillenniumproject.org/documents/maternalchild-complete.pdf*

[77] *World Health Report 2006*. World Health Organization, Geneva. Chapter 5 (Managing Exits)

[78] Department of Health and Social Security. Report on Health and Social Subjects 26: Report on confidential enquiries into maternal deaths in England and Wales 1976-1978. London: Her Majesty's Stationary Office, 1982

[79] Chalmers I, Enkin M, Keirse MJ eds. Effective care in pregnancy and childbirth 1989. Vol 1. Pregnancy. Oxford, England: Oxford University Press

[80] Ronsmans C, Filippi V. Severe obstetric morbidity. In: *Qualitative approaches for investing maternal deaths*. WHO, Geneva, 2000

[81] Promoting the use of oxytocin for the prevention of PPH Hogerzel Hans. Presented March 21,2006 at *PATH see pphprevention.org*

[82] Khan K, Wojdyla D, Say L, Gulmezoglu M, Van Look P. WHO Analysis of causes of maternal death: a systematic review. *The Lancet* 2006, 367:1066-1074

[83] Graham WJ, Bell JS and Bullough CH. Can skilled attendance at delivery reduce maternal mortality in developing countries? *Studies in Health Services Organization and Policy*, 17, 97-130

[84] Mantel G, Buchmann E, Rees H, Pattinson R. Severe Acute maternal morbidity: a pilot study of a definition of a near miss. *BJOG* Sept 1998 Vol (105) p 985

[85] Buekens P. Overmedicalization of maternal care in developing countries. *Studies in Health Services Organization and Policy*, 17, 195-206

[86] Ronsmans C. What is the evidence of the role of audits to improve the quality of obstetric care? *Studies in Health Services Organization and Policy*, 17, p 3

[87] Reducing maternal mortality in a context of poverty, Van Lerberghet W and de Brouwere V in In Safe Motherhood Strategies: a Review of the Evidence. Ed Vincent De Brouwere and Wim Van Lerberghe. *Studies in Health Services Organization and Policy*, 16, 2001, ITG Press, Belgium, 2001 p4

[88] Safe Motherhood Action Agenda: Priorities for the Next Decade; Report on Safe Motherhood Technical Consultation October 18-3, 1997 Colombo Sri Lanka. 1997, *Family Care International*

[89] Chamberlain J, Lalonde A, Arulkumaran S, McDonagh R. The role of professional associations in reducing maternal mortality worldwide. *IJGO 83* (2003) 94-102

In: Women's Health in the Majority World: Issues and Initiatives   ISBN1-1-60021-493-2
Eds: L. Elit and J. Chamberlain Froese, pp. 21-33   © 2007 Nova Science Publishers, Inc.

Chapter 2

THE TERRIBLE TRAGEDY OF NEGLECTED OBSTETRICAL CARE: FISTULA

Andrew S. Browning[1]
Barhirdar Hamlin Fistula Centre in Northern Ethiopia

ABSTRACT

Background

Obstetrical fistulas result from prolonged obstructed labor. Approximately 100,000 new cases occur annually predominantly in the developing world.

Methods

In this chapter the author discusses the presenting symptoms, associated conditions, and principles of management. Aspects of treatment and health care team training are reviewed. From the patient's perspective the social ramification are immense. However, this tragic circumstance can become an opportunity for education and rehabilitation for the affected woman.

Conclusion

The current health care resources in the developing world can only manage about 10,000 fistula repairs annually. The importance of preventing this tragedy and making resources available to rehabilitate women with fistulas is needed

---

[1] Corresponding Author: Andrew Browning MD,Barhirdar Hamlin Fistula Centre PO Box 1739,Barhirdar, Ethiopia,Email: a.s.browning@ethionet.et

OBSTETRIC FISTULA

The obstetric fistula is an age-old condition, occurring ever since women began giving birth. There is evidence of this morbidity from thousands of years ago. The mummified remain of Queen Henhenit dating from 2000BC shows a great defect between her bladder and vagina, almost certainly obstetric in origin. The first obstetric fistula to be cured was not until the mid 17th century by a Swiss physician, Yohann Fatio, but it was not until more recently, in 1855, when the world's first fistula hospital was opened in New York by the famous American gynaeocologist, James Marion Sims. He is credited with refining the techniques of surgical repair, performing 32 operations on the one woman before he succeeded in a cure. He then went on to cure many helpless women with this condition. However, his New York city fistula hospital closed over 100 years as the obstetric fistulae became extinct due to the advent of more readily available obstetric care. It then remained a forgotten condition, treated by only a handful of practitioners in remote and poor areas of the world. The condition has gained some degree of awareness recently due to the life's work of Dr Reginald and Dr Catherine Hamlin who have been treating these women in Ethiopia since 1959. Although Dr Reginald Hamlin died, Dr Catherine Hamlin is still working tirelessly in Ethiopia for these women. Their hospital has now been responsible for treating over 27,000 women with obstetric fistula in Ethiopia alone. The obstetric fistula is being treated in most countries across Africa and South East Asia. The treatment has the backing of UNFPA (United Nations Population Fund), WHO (World Health Organization) and FIGO (International Federations of Obstetricians and Gynecologists) as well as many other philanthropic organizations.

ETIOLOGY

The etiology of the obstetric fistula is clearly prolonged, unrelieved obstructed labor. During obstructed labor the presenting part is impacted against the mothers' bony pelvis and the intervening tissues suffer ischaemic necrosis if the labor is not relieved by a timely caesarean section. During the course of the labor the unborn child invariably dies after which the skull collapses and a stillborn child is delivered. The women herself is often lucky to survive and indeed if she has done so is often near to death, exhausted and often unconscious. It takes on average 26 days before she is strong enough to walk unaided [1]. However, 3-5 days after the delivery of the stillborn child, the necrotic vaginal tissue comes away exposing the fistula between her bladder and vagina and sometimes between the rectum and vagina as well. This renders the mother completely incontinent. The course of events after this is depressing. Her husband often looks after her for a time, and then, realizing that his wife is not getting better and she is indeed making the house smell and unpleasant to live in, will often divorce her. It has been noticed in Ethiopia and also in Nigeria that if a woman has had previous deliveries and live children, the husband is more likely to look after his wife and not divorce her. If however she has no living children, he is more likely to have divorced her. If so, she will return to her family who will try and care for her but likewise soon realize that their daughter or sister is not getting better and they may build a separate hut for her to dwell in. She will live in isolation. There are many anecdotal reports from Ethiopia where women with obstetric fistula have been found in huts, living alone for sometimes 10 years, rarely having ventured out for shame of her injuries and almost never having visitors due to the smell of her dwelling. Depression is of course very common as is suicidal ideation and perhaps attempts at suicide [2].

Not all fistulas are related to obstructed labor. These, although different in etiology, usually have the same social consequences. The causes include direct trauma, usually sexual, the most common cause in Ethiopia and perhaps other areas is when a child is given in marriage very young and has intercourse well before puberty. The vagina, being too small to accommodate intercourse, is either cut open, usually injuring the bladder in the process, forming a fistula, or there is direct trauma during intercourse, usually causing a tear through the perineum or a recto-vaginal fistula. In areas of war, sexual trauma can result in fistula. From a small personal series from the Democratic Republic of Congo, close to 50% of patients seen had their fistula due to rape, where there was trauma to the genital tract either with a stick, knife or bullet during the rape- ending with fistula.

Other causes of genito-urinary fistula or recto-vaginal fistula include infection- usually tuberculosis of the bladder, but there are reports or lymphogranuloma venereum. Advanced cervical cancer can present with a fistula and lastly, fistulae of the genital tract can be iatrogenic after surgery, usually a caesarean hysterectomy for ruptured uterus, or even after a hysterectomy for other gynecological ills. In cases of caesarean section it is difficult to say whether the fistula is due to the surgery or labour, as the patient will often present late in labour, up to 5 days into their labour. The fistula may already be present at the time of operation but even if it is not, the tissues at this stage of labour are edematous, even gangrenous and difficult to operate upon and a tear into the bladder may easily occur.

EPIDEMIOLOGY

The typical obstetric fistula patient is young, often below 20 years of age [1,3]. In 63% of patients the causative delivery is her first [1,4]. The average length of labour is 3.9 days following which up to 98% of women will delivery a stillborn child [1]. The typical patient is short, often less than 150cm tall and 7cm shorter than the average population [5,6,7,8]. She is poor and uneducated, 92% being illiterate [1]. On presentation over 50% of women have been divorced by their husbands, but many of the remaining are separated [9]. Most of the deliveries have been unattended and those that have been attended are usually done so by ill trained and ill equipped persons [1]. On presentation, she has been living with her condition for around 6 months (range, one week to 50 years).

PREVALENCE

No one knows for certain how many fistula patients occur each year or now many patients are waiting to be treated. There have been several hospital-based studies addressing the issue, but next to no population based studies. The WHO has stated that 0.3% of deliveries in the developing world will result in an obstetric fistula. This being the cases then there may be up to 100,000 new cases of obstetric fistula occurring each year, most of which occur in Africa. There have been other estimates of up to 500,000 cases occurring each year and up to 2 million patients waiting to be treated [10]. The worlds capacity for dealing with obstetric fistula patients remains small with an estimated 6-7000 patients being treated each year, again, mainly in Africa and the bulk of them being done by only a few dedicated surgeons.

PRESENTATION

The predominant complaint on presentation is the patients' continual and complete incontinence, but it is wrong to think of the obstetric fistula injury being just a discreet pathology occurring between the bladder and vagina. The term 'obstetric fistula injury complex' has been coined to refer to the broad range of injuries that occur during the labour [9]. The ischaemic process not only affects the tissues of the bladder and vagina and perhaps the rectum and vagina, but all the other tissues in the pelvis, the bones, muscles, nerves and the entire lower genito-urinary tract. These occur during the labour and are termed primary condition and then there are those pathologies that occur over time usually as a result of the ongoing incontinence and are termed secondary conditions.

PRIMARY CONDITIONS- THOSE RESULTING DIRECTLY FROM THE OBSTRUCTED LABOUR

Incontinence: As stated, the obvious symptom. It usually results in complete incontinence or urine and if a rectal fistula, complete flatal and faecal incontinence via the vagina. If the fistula is small, the vesico-vaginal fistula can present with symptoms similar to stress urinary incontinence, only leaking urine per vagina at times of increased intravesical pressure. Likewise if the recto-vaginal fistula is small, the patient may complain of only flatal incontinence per vaginum and perhaps incontinence of loose stool or diarrhea. Most patients only have a vesico vaginal fistula 78% while 15% have a combined recto-vaginal fistula with a vesico-vaginal fistula and only 6% have an isolated recto-vaginal fistula.[1]

Ureteric injury: In extensive obstetric fistulae, the uretero-vesical junction may be affected and the ureter may be draining straight into the vagina, away from the margin of the fistula. Sometimes the patient presents with a ureteric fistula in isolation. This usually only happens after a caesarean section performed at some stage during the obstructed labour. The patient may complain of complete urinary incontinence and also be able to void some urine normally as well as one ureter is still draining into the bladder.

Reproductive tract: The tissues of the vagina are affected and on occasion all of the vaginal tissue has been destroyed. Some 28% need some form of vaginoplasty during the repair due to severe vaginal scarring [9]. The cervix is often torn or completely split apart. Although more uncommon, vesico-uterine fistula can occur, especially if the obstruction had occurred with incomplete cervical dilation and the presenting part impinged the cervix or uterus against the pelvic brim.

Muscles of the pelvis: The levators can be affected by either direct trauma which can destroy the muscles entirely, or by causing a neuropathy.

Bones: The bony pelvis is also affected by direct trauma and ischaemia. Up to 32% show some type of abnormality on pelvic x-ray, ranging from bony spurs, areas of bony resorption to obliteration or separation of the symphysis pubis [11].

Nerves: The sacral plexus can be impinged and injured directly in the labour. Anywhere between 20-65% of patients will have some degree of foot drop [9,12]. There are other theories to its etiology, one being that during the prolonged squatting of labour, the common peroneal nerve is impinged as it traverses the head of fibula or there may be some lumbar intervertebral disc prolapse [13,14]. Several surgeons have noted that there is also some hamstring and quadriceps weakness in the affected limb reflecting either the disc prolapse of direct sacral plexus injury as the cause. Most cases of foot drop improve with time with only 13% of cases still showing signs of weakness after 2 years [12].

SECONDARY CONDITIONS-THOSE THAT RESULT AS A CONSEQUENCE OF ANY OF THE ABOVE PRIMARY CONDITIONS

Social consequences/ mental illness: In much of the developing world, there is a great deal of pressure for a woman to bear her husband children. The woman with a fistula usually has no living children and has little prospect of gaining some due to her injuries. About 52% of patients have been divorced and many of the remaining have been separated. Because of her offences she is usually shunned by her community, this combined with her embarrassment of her condition; she often lives the rest of her life in isolation. It is not surprising that many suffer depression (97%) and a significant proportion have thought about and attempted suicide [2]. The hope of an operation and then being cured certainly increases their mental health status.

Lower limb contractures: About 1-2% of patients will present with contractures of the lower extremities, usually the knee. This is due to being confined in a hut by herself for sometimes years, lying on her side in the fetal position and not walking. She can end up with not only contracture, but also severe wasting and pressure ulceration.

Upper renal tract damage: After the sloughing of the tissues from the vagina, the remaining tissue forms scar, sometimes so dense as to obliterate the vagina. The scar can obstruct the lower ureter and cause obstructive uropathies. 49% of patients can develop this and the damage can be anything from hydroureters to non-functioning kidneys [15].

Bladder stones: The patient will drink less water in an attempt to pass less urine. The resulting concentrated urine can collect in pockets in the vagina and/ or bladder and form calculi. There have been numerous instances when a traditional healer will insert some material (plant, cloth or stone) into the vagina in an attempt to stem to flow and cause a nidus for further stone formation.

Urine dermatitis: The often-concentrated urinary phosphates and nitrates continually on the skin of the perineum can cause sensitive areas of hyperkeratosis, which can also ulcerate. Secondary infections of these areas can occur.

Reproductive consequences: Up to 63% of patients will be amenorrhoeic at six months post fistula injury [9]. There are numerous reasons for this, one being neglect causing supratentorial amenorrhoea. The average BMI of patients presenting is 19 and surely many will have absent menses due to psychological strain, neglect and weight loss. A proportion will have Sheehan's syndrome from prolonged shock during the labour [16]. It is thought some will have Asherman's syndrome, likely being due to urine and infections being inside the uterus. Still more will have crypotmennorrhoea, or hidden menses as the outflow tract of cervix and vagina has been completely occluded by scar, thus the menstrual blood gets collected in the uterus causing a haematometra. Post fistula repair, the likelihood of a successful pregnancy is small. Only about 19% of repaired women will achieve a live child. If the woman does become pregnant she has a higher chance of having a miscarriage or premature delivery [17,18,19]. Many patients have a torn or split cervix from the labour and will loose their pregnancy from an incompetent cervix.

If the patient does retain her pregnancy and reach term, even with supervised vaginal deliveries, some 27% of patients will have their fistula re-opened from the delivery process [18]. Due to this it is commonly recommended that patients have an elective caesarean section at term. Some doctors recommend prolonged catheterization post elective caesarean as a precaution against any inadvertent bladder injury during dissection, which although there is no evidence, may be a prudent practice.

TREATMENT

The mainstay of treatment for obstetric fistula is surgical. Although there is a great range of different injuries and extent to the injuries in these patients and the learning curve to become a truly competent fistula surgeon is long, the basic principles of fistula surgery can be applied to all cases. These basic principles are: to protect the ureters, to mobilize widely, to have a tension free closure and to ensure a watertight closure by performing a dye test.

Only about 20% of obstetric fistula patients are easy and able to be tackled by surgeons will little experience. The remaining fistulas can be very challenging indeed with operations taking several hours. These cases may require creation of a new vagina, create a new urethra, anastomose the bladder to the urethra, reimplant the ureters into the bladder and anastomose the bowel back together. Around 15% of recto-vaginal fistulae need a temporary diverting colostomy before the operation if the rectal injury is large, high and/or extensively scarred.

Post-operatively the recovery time is about 2 weeks. The bladder needs to be kept completely empty with continuous catheter drainage for 14 days. If the bladder fills with urine during this time, then pressure can be placed on the repair and disrupt the sutures leading to a breakage and failure of the operation. It needs vigilant nursing care to ensure that the patients is drinking enough to irrigate the bladder with dilute urine and ensure that there are no blockages in the catheter drainage system. The patients can be educated to notice if there is a blockage in the flow of urine, but this should not be relied upon without good nursing backup. The 2-week post-operative hospitalization is difficult for many centers where hospital beds are few and to have one patients occupying one bed for so long can be a strain on the hospital system. It does not appear that a shorter hospital stay is possible without compromising patient outcome. Nor is it possible for the patient to go home with the catheter as many patients have to travel for some days to get home including many hours if not days walk. This combined with often-limited access to drinking water whilst at home and very limited hygiene makes this not an option.

The outcomes of surgery can be variable. It is possible with experience to be able to close almost any fistula that a surgeon is faced with, with closure rates of up to 92-96% with the first operation being boasted. This does not however equate with a cure as many will have incontinence even with the fistula closed, the reason being that most of the mechanisms that are normally in place to maintain urinary and faecal incontinence in a women have been destroyed during the labour and there is very little tissue left from which to reconstruct them. Up to 33% of patients still have urinary incontinence post repair that can be so severe that the patient feels that the operation has completely failed [20]. It is thought that some of those patients with more mild incontinence will improve with time as the bladder gets accustomed to holding urine again. One surgeon in northern Nigeria has followed his patients for 6 months post repair and he claimed that upon catheter removal post repair, about 33% of patients do have incontinence per urethra, but after 6 months, this figure has reduced to 15%. (Waaldjik, personal communication).

After treatment the patient is taught that she should abstain from sexual contact for 3 months and if she does become pregnant she should go to a hospital at about 7 months pregnant and wait nearby having her antenatal checks until it is time for her antenatal check.

THE INOPERABLE FISTULA

There are a number of obstetric fistulae that are so extensive that a cure is simply impossible. It is almost always possible to cure a recto-vaginal fistula, but if a vesico-vaginal fistula is so extensive to have had destroyed most if not all of the bladder tissue, continence per urethra is almost impossible. The only way to make these patients continent and then have any quality of life is to perform a urinary diversion operation. The two more commonly used operations are the Mainz II pouch; diverting the urine into a pouch of sigmoid and thus the urine is passed per rectum. This needs a continent anal sphincter to contain the liquid faeces/ urine that is passed and many patients will leak some faeces/ urine at night when the sphincter relaxes. The other option is an ileal conduit. This needs ongoing specialized equipment, which is not readily available in most centers. Even if the conduit bags are available, it is usually only in one or two locations and hence the patient is unable to return to her village to live, but ends up living in or close by to the institution that performed the operation. The Addis Ababa Fistula Hospital has built a village near the hospital where these incurable patients will live together.

TREATMENT ISSUES

There are a hopelessly inadequate number of institutions that perform fistula surgery given the numbers needed to meet the demand. There are a number of reasons for this. One is that the condition occurs in areas of poverty, in areas of poor medical resources. It is also a condition of poverty in that the patient is often destitute, unable to raise the money needed for treatment and sometimes unable to even to raise the money to cover the transport costs to a hospital.

Most fistula patients are treated for free and because of this it is mainly missions, NGO's (Non-Governmental Organizations) and charities. There are of course some treated in the local government hospitals, and, although sometimes they are treated for free, the inability of these patients to pay limits the number of patients treated in this way. Many institutions have found ways to make the cost of treating these patients very low indeed and the range of treatment costs varies depending on the available resources of the institution.

The staffs themselves have to be dedicated and compassionate. The work in treating these patients is immensely satisfying in that when the when cured the patients are incredibly grateful. However there is very little monetary reward and the people involved are usually altruistic. The auxiliary staff also have to be very dedicated. Fistula units contain several if not hundreds of completely incontinent women as they wait for treatment. The floors, bedclothes and patient gowns need to be washed several times a day to keep the odor at bay. In Addis Ababa this problem has been solved by employing fistula patients to be the nursing aids and cleaners and laundry workers. These employees are usually patients who, due to the severity of their injuries cannot be totally cured and there is no hope of them returning home to rejoin their families and societies. They are grateful for the opportunity to work and have a role and be cared for within the institution. They make exceptional nursing aids as they know exactly what it is to have been through the ordeal of the long labour, the shame of the resulting incontinence and the fear and apprehension of coming to a hospital for the first time. They take time to talk to the patients, to explain and put them to ease.

There are also questions of where is best to treat these patients. Some are treated within the confines of a larger general hospital. This works well but there are some drawbacks. This means that the patient is placed in a general surgical or gynecological ward with other general patients. From experience from several centers, this has proved difficult as the other patients and staff are often not so sympathetic towards them and some patients have even been forced to leave the ward by the other patients on account of their smell. She is deeply ashamed of her injuries and being with other women or patients without this condition can be emotionally difficult.

The next option is to treat the obstetric fistula patient in a separate ward within the general hospital. This model has been replicated across the world with some success. It has the advantage of being able to care for these women together, which has psychological advantages. It also has the advantage that the staff will be better accustomed to dealing with these patients and more sensitive to their needs. The little ward will be dependant upon the other resources of the hospital, the theatres, the laboratory, pharmacy, laundry and kitchen. In times of great demand for the operating theatre, the obstetric fistula patient might be placed lower on the waiting list for operation as her condition is of a chronic nature, not acute. There may also be constraints on the physician in charge of these patients. The physician is usually a gynecologist or general surgeon and he interested may be stretched with demands from the general hospital.

The final option is to build an entirely independent fistula unit. This has the advantages of negating the above conflicts of interest that may occur in a general hospital, but it has the disadvantages of being much more expensive to run as the hospital will have to have its own administration, theatres, laboratory, pharmacy, laundry, kitchen and auxiliary staff. It will also have to raise its own money as these centers are usually entirely charitable, not dependant on paying patients or a government budget and a lot of time and energy is expended in raising the necessary funds to carry out treatment.

There are many patients who are treated by the way of 'fistula camps'. This is when a visiting surgeon is invited to hospital to treat a number of fistula patients 'on bloc'. Usually an operating table is reserved for this and all other elective operation lists are suspended for the one or two weeks of the camp. The patients come by means of advertising by radio or by information dispersing via health center and village elders. It is an opportunity for training for the local physicians in obstetric fistula management and surgery.

TRAINING ISSUES

Currently there are only 2 institutions that provide ongoing training in fistula surgery, in northern Nigeria and Ethiopia. Demand is high for training and as yet, both places only train people to repair the basic or simple fistula. The training occurs over one month and the trainee is expected to first observe, then assist and finally perform operation himself or herself as well as being involved in the pre-operative and post-operative care of the patients in the hospital. The waiting list is for the training is long. The trainees are usually from an NGO (Non Governmental Organization) or mission involved in charity or governmental hospital that is already caring for fistula patients. It is anticipated that after the completion of the training the trainee will be competent in the straight forward fistula and will have the an understanding of the basic principles of fistula repair and over time build upon those skills to be able to undertake more difficult cases. It is important that the novice in fistula surgery should know their limits and not undertake cases beyond their limits. The main reason for this is this increases the chance of a breakdown of repair which is not only discouraging to the patient but also the surgeon and it makes the second attempt of repair more difficult. Some centers boast of a 94% success rate in closing a fistula at the first attempt, but if this fails the success at subsequent operations decrease rapidly to 73% at the second operation and 51% for the third attempt.

The other option for training is at 'fistula camps' when a visiting surgeon visits a hospital to perform an intensive 1 or 2 weeks of fistula surgery. The local surgeons are trained intensively over the time of the camp. The surgeon often visits the same center once or twice a year and provides further training and so with time, the local surgeons are trained in more and more difficult cases. This also has the advantage that the surgeon is trained in their own environment and equipment and also the whole team in theatre and ward are trained.

SOCIAL ISSUES

The women who sustain an obstetric fistula are from the poorest areas of the world. These women usually have had no education, have little power or position and one of their main roles in life is to bear children. If she has failed to do so and has also sustained terrible ostracizing injuries there is little hope for her to have any sort of quality of life. She has invariably been divorced or separated. Her injuries and offenses make it impossible for her to engage in normal social circles- she is usually too ashamed to want to socialize with others and others will not want to come close for fear of her condition and the smell. She will live in isolation with no care and no hope. Depression is of course high as is suicidal ideation, and cases of suicide attempts and successful suicide attempts have been reported. In any fistula unit, there is a high degree of camaraderie amongst the patients and Dr Hamlin of the Addis Ababa Fistula Hospital, Ethiopia calls it the 'sisterhood of suffering'. Certainly this fellowship goes a long way to their mental healing. Some fistula centres have full time counselors and even some counselors who are available to return to the fistula patients village with them after they are cured. Most centres do not have the resources for such a service and concentrate more upon the patients physical healing and not their mental healing. It should always be remembered that these patients have been through a terrible amount of suffering, losing their child, the trauma of the prolonged labour itself, the loss of their dignity, friends, husband and family and social responsibilities.

REHABILITATION

There are a number of physical rehabilitation issues that need to be address. As stated a number of patients will have difficulty with mobility from foot drop and also from contractures of the lower limbs. Again, where obstetric fistula patients present, it is in areas of poor resources and poor medical facilities. Physiotherapy is the mainstay of treatment for issues of immobility, but if the contractures of the lower limbs are severe, then it can take months before she is mobile again- a difficult patient for the average resource poor hospital to accommodate.

The pelvic floor muscles also need to be rehabilitated. One small unpublished series by the author showed that in obstetric fistula patients there is a decreasing power in the pelvic floor muscles the lower the fistula is in the genitor-urinary tract. This may also influence the higher incidence of stress urinary incontinence in women with fistulae involving the urethra. Pelvic floor muscle exercises ('Kegel exercises') should be taught to all obstetric fistula patients with lower injuries and they should be educated in the value of continuing them long into the future as there are many anecdotal cases of patients with stress urinary incontinence post fistula repair who, after some months of pelvic floor exercises improve and become continent again.

Many patients also require, sometimes intensive, nutritional rehabilitation. As stated the average BMI (body mass index) of patients presenting to the Addis Ababa Fistula Hospital is 19, but some are much less and present with hypoproteinaemia. They need high protein diets and regular weighing until they are in a fit state to be operated upon.

EDUCATION

The patients on arrival are in hospital for a minimum of 2 weeks, as the bladder needs to be kept on free drainage for 2 weeks post fistula repair. In reality, she is admitted to hospital for much longer for different forms of rehabilitation and also waiting time prior to a space in the operation list. It is a valuable opportunity to educate the women on various topics from hygiene, sanitation, health, diet, even some basic literacy. There are also programmes in some centers to educate the women on their legal rights as they pertain to their particular country. It is often the only education that the patient has ever received and the opportunity should not be missed. Having said this, in Addis Ababa, Ethiopia, there is an education programme in place, part of which is to educate the woman on how her injury actually occurred, that is due to the obstructed labour. A recent survey on discharge found that many women still not fully understand the association between her long labour and the occurrence of the fistula. They often still thought that the incontinence was due to a bad spirit or due to some medical manipulation received during the labour. One has to be careful how it is explained and the education brought across.

THE FUTURE

There are embarrassingly few places that are treating obstetric fistula in any number. It has been estimated that there are at least 2 million patients with obstetric fistula still waiting for treatment, mainly across Africa, but currently the world's capacity for dealing with the problem stands at about 6000-7000 cases being done per year. There should be a referral center for the treatment of these women in each area of Africa and this should also act as a training center for that region. The referral center should act as a support for the other hospitals within that region with respect to further training for the regional staff and quality control. However, the main target for the future should be towards prevention of this condition.

Obstetric fistula is a forgotten condition in the western world simply because it is safely preventable with the availability of good obstetric care. If all women had monitoring during their labour and then prompt access to medical assistance if needed, it would not only go towards preventing obstetric fistulae, but also save countless lives of women and their babies during childbirth. However, the task towards this is immense. It has been estimated that if obstetric fistulae were to be prevented across Africa, then 75,000 new obstetric units would have to be built [21]. That would not only mean that medical staff would have to be trained and employed to maintain these centers, but also the communities would have to be educated about the value of antenatal care, the value of intrapartum care and safe delivery. There would also have to be the manpower in the villages to enable the antenatal care and education. Roads would have to be built to enable safe transport to an obstetric unit; money would have to be raised for the communities and families to be able to transport their women. Communications systems would need to be in place for referral and transport. Reducing maternal morbidity and mortality is one of the millennium development goals and money needs to be in place to at least start to care for and treat pregnant women. Due to the immensity of this task some more novel approaches have been implemented in some regions, for example, the use of maternity waiting areas around hospitals where high-risk pregnant women can go a wait for their delivery from about 36 weeks pregnant. They are monitored antenatally and if there should be complications during their labour that needs attention, then they are at the hospital already. Africa has a chronic shortage of doctors. Many qualified doctors leave their countries in hope of a better life somewhere else, leaving fewer and fewer people behind. One remedy for this problem is to train health officers in emergency obstetric care and build their skills so that they can diagnose the need for and then perform caesarean section. This has several advantages in that it is quicker and cheaper to train these professionals and the nature of their qualification is such that it is more difficult for them to immigrate to another country and find employment there.

It is unfortunate that in this day and age the world still has an immensely high maternal morbidity and mortality rate and obstetric fistula is still relatively common. Hopefully with more attention to this condition the world may go some way towards it eradication. This is a long and distant dream for the future, in the meantime we still need to care for and treat the victims of the neglected labour.

KEY POINTS

- Obstetrical fistulas occur as a result of prolonged unrelieved obstructed labor
- The primary condition includes, urinary incontinence, possible injury to ureter(s), pelvic floor muscle, and nerve (including drop foot)
- Secondary issues include the social consequences such as divorce, living in isolation and depression; bladder stones and urine dermatitis
- The treatment is surgical, rehabilitation and education
- The future involves improving obstetrical care to intervene early in obstructed labor and prevent the tissue ischemia that leads to the fistula.

REFERENCES

[1]   Kelly, J; Kwast, BE. Epidaemiological study of vesico-vaginal fistulas in Ethiopia. *Int Urol J,* 1993 4, 278-281.
[2]   Goh, JTW; Sloane, KM; Krause, HG; Browning, A; Akhter, S. Mental health screening in women with genital tract fistulae. *Br J Obstet Gynaecol,* Sept 2005 112(9), 1328-30.
[3]   Tahzib, F. Epidemiological determinants of vesicovaginal fistulas. *Br J Obstet Gynaecol,* 1983 90, 387-391.
[4]   Danso, KA; Martley, JO; Wall, LL. The epidemiology of genitourinary fistulae in Kumasi, Ghana 1977-1992. *Int Urogyn J,* 1996 7, 117-120.
[5]   Wall, LL; Karshima, JA; Kirschner, C; *et al.* The obstetric vesicovaginal fistula: Characteristics of 899 patients from Jos, Nigeria. *Amer J of Obstets and Gyn,* 2004 190, 1011-1019.
[6]   Bhasker Rao, K. Genital fistula. *J of Obstet and Gynae of India,* 1975 25, 58-65.
[7]   Bal, JS. The vesico-vaginal and allied fistulae- a report on 40 cases. *Med J of Zambia,* 1975 9, 69-71.
[8]   Ampofo, K; Out, T; Uchebo, G. Epidaemiology of vesico-vaginal fistulae in northern Nigeria. *West African J of Med,* 1990 9, 98-102.
[9]   Arrowsmith, S; Hamlin, EC; Wall, LL. Obstructed labour injury complex: Obstetric fistula formation and the multifaceted morbidity of maternal birth trauma in the developing world. *Obstet and Gynaecol Survey,* 1996 51, 568-574.
[10]   Waaldjik, K. The immediate management of fresh obstetric fistulas with catheter and/ or early closure. *Int J Gynaecol and Obstet,* 1994 45, 11-16.

[11] Cockshott, WP. Pubic changes associated with obstetric vesico-vaginal fistulae. *Clinical Radiology,* 1973 24, 241-247.

[12] Waaldjik, K; Elkins, TE. The obstetric fistula and peroneal nerve injury: an analysis of 974 consecutive patients. *Int Urogynaecol J,* 1994 5, 12-14.

[13] Reif, ME. Bilateral common peroneal nerve palsy secondary to prolonged squatting in natural childbirth. *Birth,* 1988 15, 100-102.

[14] Sinclair, RSC. Maternal obstetric palsy. *South African Med J,* 1952 26, 708-714.

[15] Langundoye, SB; Bell, D; Gill, G; *et al.* Urinary changes in obstetric vesico-vaginal fistulae: a report of 216 cases studied by intravenous urography. *Clinical Radiology,* 1972 27, 531-539.

[16] Bieler, RW; Schnabel, T. Pituitary and ovarian function in women with vesicovaginal fistula after obstructed and prolonged labour. *South African Med J,* 1976 50, 257-266.

[17] Aimaku, VE. Reproductive functions after the repair of obstetric vesicovaginal fistulae. *Fertility and Sterility,* 1974 25, 586-591.

[18] Evoh, NJ; Akinia, O. Reproductive performance after the repair of obstetric vesico-vaginal fistulae. *Annals of Clinical Research,* 1978 10, 303-306.Bhasker Rao, K. Vesicovaginal fistula- a study of 269 cases. *J Obstet Gynae India,* 1972 22, 536-541.

[19] Browning, A; Prevention of residual urinary stress incontinence following successful repair of obstetric vesico-vaginal fistula using a fibro-muscular sling. *Br J Obstet Gynaecol,* 2004 111, 357-361.

[20] Waaldik, K; *Evaluation report XIV on VVF projects in Northern Nigeria and Niger,* Katsin, Nigeria: Babbar Ruga Fistula Hospital; 1998.

In: Women's Health in the Majority World: Issues and Initiatives   ISBN1-1-60021-493-2
Eds: L. Elit and J. Chamberlain Froese, pp. 35-48   © 2007 Nova Science Publishers, Inc.

Chapter 3

IF WOMEN COUNTED: THE ROLE OF SKILLED BIRTH ATTENDANTS IN SURVEILLANCE OF MATERNAL DEATHS

Ann Montgomery[1]

Ontario, Canada and Nepal

ABSTRACT

Millennium Development Goal number five (MDG-5) sets the target that by 2015, maternal mortality ratio will be reduced three-quarters. This is to be done by increasing the proportion of skilled birth attendants providing care in an enabling environment. However, measuring where we are now, and where we will be in 2015 is extremely difficult, if not impossible, because the majority of the women who die, do so in an area of the world with inadequate surveillance or death registration. Efforts to address the difficulty of counting women who die at home, en route to hospital or once in hospital have had mixed success. Efforts to derive a best guess are commonly used though provide a large error range, making before-and-after comparisons inaccurate. Obstetric service indicators are now proposed as a means of measuring whether or not service is adequate, without the effort of counting the women, but this method has yet to be properly evaluated and there may be limitations when this method is transplanted to different settings. Worldwide, skilled birth attendants play an integral role in not only attaining MDG-5, but ensuring we have the numbers to demonstrate that we have truly arrived. As the increase in skilled birth attendants converges with the hoped for decrease in the maternal mortality ratio, a system of counting has to be in place to ensure that women's lives are being saved.

[1] Corresponding Author: Email: annlmontgomery@yahoo.ca

ESTIMATING THE GLOBAL MATERNAL MORTALITY RATIO

In 1985, the World Health Organization (WHO) produced the first "guestimate" that half a million women were dying each year due to complications related to reproduction, and 99% of these deaths were occurring in developing countries. With this new understanding of the magnitude of the problem, in 1987, Nairobi hosted the Safe Motherhood Conference, sponsored by WHO, UNFPA and the World Bank—this lead to the launch of the Safe Motherhood Initiative (SMI) [2]. In 1994, the International Conference on Population and Development (ICPD) in Cairo rejuvenated the SMI agenda and member states set the goal to reduce maternal mortality by half by 2000, and by a further half by 2015. At the ICPD+5 in 1999, the international community reaffirmed the goals of the SMI and agreed that maternal mortality should be used as an indicator of efforts to strengthen health systems [3]. Then in 2000, the Millennium Declaration was endorsed by 189 countries. Stating in Millennium Development Goal Number 5 (MDG-5), it called for a three-quarter reduction of maternal deaths worldwide by 2015, to be met by increasing the proportion of skilled attendance at delivery.

However, the maternal mortality "guestimate" produced by the WHO for 1990, 1995, and 2000 is not accurate enough to measure short term, worldwide trends [1,4,5]. Nor is it precise enough to allow for country-to-country comparisons. Also, the methodology to arrive at the estimate in 1990 is slightly different than the methodology used in 2000, making the before-and-after comparison problematic. Yet, this is the proxy measure chosen to evaluate attainment of the MGD-5; the state of a country's health care system, specifically, the delivery of health care to women. The paradox being that the regions of the world with the highest estimated maternal morality ratios also have no system of surveillance.

According to the WHO, in *Maternal Mortality in 2000* (*http://www.who.int/reproductive-health/publications/maternal_mortality_2000/mme.pdf*, Accessed June 14, 2006), of the 60 countries with good death registration and good cause of death records (1% of estimated maternal deaths), one is in Africa (Mauritius), and two are in Asia (Mongolia, Singapore). Forty-seven per cent of the estimated maternal deaths occur in Africa, and 48% in Asia. So in regions with the highest number of maternal deaths, and the highest maternal mortality ratio, the calculated estimate relies on surveys or calculations from mathematical models. For 51 countries (61% of estimated maternal deaths), the maternal mortality ratio was calculated from surveys, adjusted based on the validity of the survey used. For 62 countries (38% of maternal deaths), a mathematical model is used which takes into account the country's fertility rate, proportion of deliveries attended by skilled health personnel, contraceptive availability, status of women, gross domestic product, and two indicator variables—one defining the region under study and the one signifying the completeness of adult death registration [1]. This method gives a large range of error (not confidence intervals in the strict statistical sense). For example, the range of error in the maternal mortality ratio, per 100 000 live births, for Afghanistan (470 to 3500), Burundi (260 to 1900), Cote d'Ivoire (170 to 1300), Guinea-Bissau (280 to 2100), Liberia (190 to 1400), and Tanzania (910 to 2200) are so large, that they cannot be used to measure trends in the country or region, nor can they be used to provide comparisons between time or place.

Estimation exercises such as this can draw attention to the issue by providing simple answers for mass media distribution, for what is a complex social issue. It does not sufficiently shame governments into action, as governments can dismiss the figures as inaccurate. It does, however, debase the MDG agenda by setting out a goal that is impossible to measure.

IMPROVING THE ESTIMATION OF MATERNAL MORTALITY RATIO

In countries such as Canada, US and Europe, under-reporting and misclassification occur despite vital registry systems, universal medical certification, and relative ease of access to autopsy and case investigation [6,7]. Studies in individual countries to audit and validate the reporting methodology needs to be undertaken in an effort to determine the rate of under-reporting and misclassification and calculate the appropriate adjustment factor to be applied to national maternal mortality ratio. Studies such as these should look at efforts to capture maternal deaths (searching multiple sources of information), and attempts to confirm maternal deaths with confidential enquiries.

Routine surveillance is done using district health surveys (DHS) and vital registration (*http://www.who.int/reproductive-health/publications/maternal_mortality_2000/mme.pdf,* Accessed June 14, 2006). This type of surveillance is not meant to characterize the maternal death, and often misses the poorest, most underserved population. One-time research studies to measure MMR are the sisterhood method, RAMOS, and cross-sectional studies. The sisterhood method is retrospective, looking back ten years to estimate the number of maternal deaths by interviewing the sisters of women who have died during the childbearing years (e.g, 12-45 years)—while it is quick and inexpensive, it cannot give a reflection of change due to an intervention. RAMOS—reproductive age mortality study—identifies and investigates the deaths of all women of reproductive age. Deaths are identified by informants and records (civil registers, hospitals, health centres, community leaders, school children, religious authorities, undertakers, cemetery officials). It does not provide an accurate estimate of MMR unless there is accurate registration of the number of live births (the denominator). Cross-sectional studies are used by many developed countries in which the number of maternal deaths is counted from vital registration. Figure 1 illustrates the breakdown in the methodology used for the derivation of the MMR estimates in the latest WHO report.

Methodology for systematic reviews of observational studies in maternal mortality and morbidity is in its infancy in an effort to identify variables that would further assist in calculating estimates of maternal mortality in areas without vital registration [8].

In the only systematic review to date, the UN group included studies that reported prevalence/incidence of maternal mortality reported after 1990, contained a sample size greater than 200 and a clear description of the methodology. From the included studies, they extracted information about the population and setting, maternal mortality measure, the definition of maternal death used, and whether researchers made efforts to capture all the maternal deaths. They looked for associations between the maternal mortality ratio and specific national demographics: infant mortality rate, proportion of births attended by skilled birth attendants, contraceptive-use prevalence rate, health expenditure per capita and female net primary school enrolment ratio. By examining 141 countries, they were able to capture a sample of 78% of the global births—a limitation of the study was lack of data from China. Contraceptive-use prevalence rate and female net primary school enrolment ratio were not statistically significant (i.e. show no association with the maternal mortality ratio regionally), and a positive association with infant mortality rate, and a negative association with proportion of births attended by a skilled birth attendant and health expenditure per capita were statistically significant.

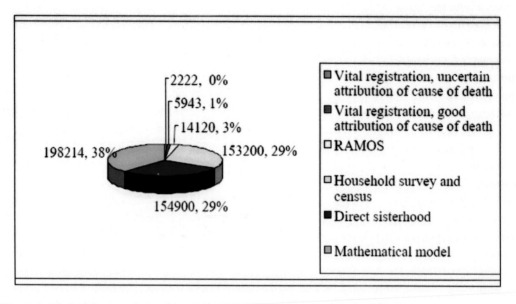

Figure 1. Methodology to derive the estimated number of maternal death, 2000 [1].

WHY DO WOMEN DIE?

Missing the mark on the MDG-5 aside, simply understanding that many women are dying because they are women, and improving the situation so that so many women do not die, is the goal. Since the issue of maternal deaths is one of eight MGDs, it is evident we recognize that maternal deaths are unique, and occur in sufficient numbers to justify efforts and resources to improve the situation. However, the circular argument is "How will we know if we have improved the situation if we cannot accurately count the number of women dying?" The current idea is not to count the women but rather to count the availability and distribution of obstetric service indicators. This is done for children where vaccination coverage is counted more easily than measles cases, and oral-rehydration uptake is counted more easily than diarrhoeal cases.

Lack of Skilled Attendant at Delivery

A skilled birth attendant refers exclusively to "people with midwifery skills (for example, doctors, midwives, nurses) who have been trained to proficiency in the skills necessary to manage normal deliveries and diagnose or refer obstetric complications, excluding trained and untrained Traditional Birth Attendants" (*http://www.who.int/reproductive-health/publications/2004/skilled_attendant.pdf*, Access June 14, 2006) [9].

Evidence supporting the association of skilled birth attendance on reducing maternal mortality comes from historic and contemporary studies in developed countries, and the WHO systematic study mentioned above, yet all studies are confounded by level of development of pooled country data, education, and the enabling environment in which the skilled birth attendant works [10-13].

Swedish evidence is found in unique 19th and 20th century parish records. Legislation passed by politicians, local medical officials using nascent theories of public health, and the training of midwives with follow-up contact for dissemination of recommended clinical protocols. An important factor is when public health officials reinforced the importance of handwashing and instrument sterilization with carbolic soap supported the continued decreasing trend in puerperal sepsis in 1890 at midwifery attended births. This is in contrast to the increase in puerperal sepsis at the same time in the UK, where midwifery and medical men were not working together but rather in contrast to one another [10]. Sweden also provides an early example of professional back-up support for complicated cases arising at midwifery-attended home deliveries [14]. The MMR in Sweden in 1881 was 228 per 100 000 live births. Netherlands, Denmark and Norway went on to adopt similar policies and experienced similar success in a reduction of maternal deaths whereas the United States did not, and the number of maternal deaths remained high. The exception to this is the Frontier Nursing Service, in 1935-37 reported a MMR of 66. Following the introduction of antibiotics, caesarean deliveries, and blood transfusions, between the 1937 and 1970, the maternal mortality ratio dropped in the US and Sweden to 10 per 100 000 live births where it has remained [15].

A contemporary example in the United States involving the *absence* of skilled attendance is found in a cloistered religious group, in which literate well-nourished women experienced 6 maternal deaths for 344 live births (2 due to sepsis, and 4 due to postpartum hemorrhage)—in the complete absence of prenatal, intrapartum or postpartum care. From this small sample, the MMR extrapolates to 872 per 100 000 [16]. A contemporary example of *introducing* improvement with skilled attendance at delivery in Jamaican rural areas, and improvement in transportation to hospital which corresponded with a decline in the maternal mortality ratio [17].

All skilled birth attendants must have core midwifery skills (http//www. *internationalmidwives.org/modules.php?op=modloadandname=Newsandfile=articleandsid= 27* , Accessed June 14, 2006). A joint statement by the International Confederation of Midwives, the International Federation of Gynecology and Obstetrics, and the WHO recommends national regulation and licensing of skilled attendants, in order to protect the public, ensuring that re-accreditation and re-licensing mechanisms to improve quality of care (e.g. continuing education, re-accreditation schemes, and supervision models). As well as the training institution and workplaces need to be nationally licensed and regulated [9].

We understand the value of the role that skilled birth attendants have in care for women at all stages of pregnancy and postpartum [18], however, questions have been raised regarding the use of the number of skilled birth attendants as a proxy measure for estimating maternal deaths.

Poor care delivered by skilled attendants could increase the number of maternal deaths. When SBAs are separated into number of doctors versus MMR, and midwives versus MMR, the number of doctors corresponds to an L-shape graph where a small increase in the number of doctors corresponds to a sharp decrease in the MMR. Conversely, there is no linear or otherwise association between the number of midwives and the MMR. This is likely due to the varied definition of the role and status of midwives internationally [19]. As well, including doctors in the number of skilled attendants does not reflect their role in the delivery and possibly, their absence in the monitoring and management of the labour and post-partum period. The core midwifery skills reflect midwifery training and not obstetric training.

Using the number of skilled birth attendants may reflect the number of women who can afford skilled attendance and not the number of women who need skilled attendance. And finally, the number of skilled attendants does not reflect the care needed by women encountering life-threatening events outside the point of delivery (i.e. ectopic pregnancy, spontaneous and induced abortion, late post-partum haemorrhage, and post-partum depression and psychosis).

There is still a need for evidence that the number of skilled birth attendants can act as a useful proxy measure for estimating MMR.

Lack of Emergency Obstetric Care

It is well recognised that if the skilled attendant is to be of any use, there is to be access to emergency obstetric care. What constitutes emergency obstetric care has been laid out by the WHO. Service indicators of 4 basic and 1 comprehensive emergency obstetric care facility per 500 000 population. A basic emergency obstetric care facility has intravenous anti-hemorrhagic meds, antibiotics, and anti-convulsant meds; can perform manual removal of the placenta and remove retained placental products; and can perform forceps or vacuum delivery. Comprehensive emergency obstetric facility can provide basic emergency obstetric care, caesarean delivery and blood transfusions [20] (*http://www.who.int/reproductive-health/publications/rh_indicators/guidelines.pdf* , Access June 14 , 2006). It is important to cautiously interpret this because the existence of the equipment and the theoretical knowledge of staff does not necessary translate into appropriate, timely intervention.

Lack of Political Will

Knowing how many women are dying is a very important point when drumming up international support and political will. In a case study of Indonesia from 1987-1997, four factors were highlighted on how to generate political will to lower maternal mortality in resource-poor settings. These are the existence of clear indicators showing that a problem exists, the presence of effective political entrepreneurs to push the cause, the organization of attention-generating focus events to promote widespread concern for the issue, and the availability of politically palatable policy alternatives that enable national leaders to understand that the problem is surmountable [21].

The WHO systematic study did find a relationship between estimated MMR and health expenditure per capital [13]. Whereas a previous study found a sharp L-shaped curve where the estimated maternal mortality ratio drops from very high to very low with a small increase in health expenditure per capita and does not drop substantially with greater and greater expenditure[22]. Using 1990s data, Vietnam, Lesotho, Central African Republic and Nepal all had similar purchasing power with MMR estimate of 160, 600, 700 and 1500 respectively

[15]. There is still much research to be done in determining what are the best, cost-effective interventions. Initiative for Maternal Mortality Programme Assessment (IMMPACT) is a research initiative to examine evidence-based cost-effective strategies to lower maternal mortality (*http://www.abdn.ac.uk/immpact/index.php* , Accessed June 14, 2006).

WHAT IS THE ROLE OF SBAS IN MATERNAL MORTALITY SURVEILLANCE

Improved Data Quality

In many regions, the act of surveillance seems trivial when there are so many other facets of obstetric care yet to be put in place. In places where homes have no address, communities have no health care system, and Ministries of Health have small budgets, it is impossible to accurately count the number of women dying from pregnancy-related complications. In countries with vital registrations, census data, and large healthcare budgets, counting the number of women dying, which is very small, is also difficult to accurately assess.

However, the position of the skilled birth attendant is optimal for counting women. And with the introduction of more and more SBAs, their role in surveillance should not be overlooked.

Worldwide, there is a staggering amount of unanalyzed and uninterpreted information. As clinicians, we produce massive amounts of documentation, and rarely turn-around to reflect on the information we produce. The data is often left in storage because we do not fully acknowledge its value, and therefore do not set aside time to evaluate it. The data are routine, and not highly valued by researchers due to lack of standardization and many errors.

Every clinician and facility keeps a variety of documentation. The quality of record-keeping and documentation varies but is rarely complete. Tools for improving documentation are site specific, but have to take into account the needs and abilities of staff. The demonstrated strength of the partograph, [23], for example, are not yet fully realized by many clinicians—and training in this area still needs to be provided. Charting-by-exception is a tool utilizing tick boxes to save time, provides reassurance for normal events and identifies abnormal—as well as providing monitoring reminders for clinicians. A database search found no studies applying this charting in resource-poor setting.

There is also often the overlooked need to standardize the language in which clinicians document (usually the language of the old colonizer or the preferred language of training for potential emigrants is adopted)—this practice should be questioned as narrative notes are not recorded in the language in which the clinician is most fluent and therefore limited, incomplete, or absent—notes in the preferred language of the clinician are better than no notes.

For clinicians to fully appreciate the value of quality documentation, the chart has to be put into use: giving the clinicians the opportunity to return to the notes to re-evaluate their management, facilitating transfer of care to another clinician, and a historical record of the outcomes of care provided by this clinician and her or his team.

Peer Review

Clinicians are not motivated to provide excellent documentation if their documentation is never reviewed. Peer-review is a confidential process in which peers review cases together (*http://www.aom.on.ca/files/Office_Documents/Communications/No_3_-_Practice_Guide_to _Peer_Review_updated.doc* , Accessed June 14, 2006). They do so in a supportive, non-threatening environment with the aim of learning and providing better care. Peer-review provides an opportunity for more experienced clinicians to discuss cases with new clinicians and students. It provides an opportunity to present the textbook information and new research as it pertains to a presented case.

It can allow for a multi-disciplinary framework, however, in the majority of settings, midwives and nurses are not peers with but rather subordinates to doctors and therefore, there own peer review process can allow them to develop and foster autonomy, which can improve their confidence, sense of responsibility and competence in their role as the primary care providers. Peer review can also be used as a forum to seek advice regarding management of an on-going case. Students benefit by participating in and presenting their own cases at peer-review. There are intangible benefits in which relationships develop that would not otherwise (e.g. clinicians working opposite shifts, clinicians working in the community and facility), and establishing inter-facility peer-review can foster relationships between rural and urban, or primary and referral centers.

Clinicians can decide on the frequency of peer-reviews (e.g. 6 to 12 per year) and the number of cases to be reviewed. The group may decide on mandatory cases to be reviewed such as maternal and perinatal deaths and cases of morbidity or 'near-misses', and require that these cases be reviewed in a timely fashion (e.g. within 48 hours). The clinician(s) then has (have) 48 hours to ensure that the documentation is complete, adding late entries as necessary[2], and completing vital registration forms. The group may wish to invite review of rare or interesting cases as well.

If the time is set aside for peer-review, not all cases may be reviewed in the allotted time, conversely, if there are no cases for review, then a random chart is pulled to review. The point is that there are short, regular intervals protected for review and reflection of past cases. Time for attendance is the only direct cost of peer-review.

No notes are taken during peer-review, only the names of those in attendance and any recommendations put forward are recorded. In some jurisdictions, peer-review attendance is a requirement for ongoing registration or licensing. If this is not the case, the facility may consider making it a requirement for employment or issuing privileges.

Even the best clinicians can become complacent and provide substandard care. This is illustrated in studies in which surveyed staff have good awareness of best practice but do not always put this understanding into practice [24] (*http://www.who.int/reproductive-health/publications/btn/text.pdf*, Accessed June 14, 2006). Peer-review, especially in the absence of a punitive medico-legal framework, provides clinicians with some motivation to complete the chart, present their management for review, defend their actions, provides them with an opportunity to ask for support and guidance, and as a group, they can make

---

[2] A late entry is recorded in the chart. The clinician records the date and time that the entry is made, and then provides the date, approximate time and details of the event that was not entered contemporaneously in the chart.

recommendations for improvements in care. While peer-review is ideally non-threatening, confidential, and supportive, with the aim to learn from cases to improve care—persistent negligence on the part of a clinician requires disciplinary action with the involvement of the regulatory body of the profession.

Sometimes, there are no recommendations following peer-review. Confidentiality should foster honesty, and recognition that clinicians make mistakes or could have made better decisions—this should lead to meaningful recommendations that staff will feel committed to implementing. Recommendations should focus on actions that the clinicians can undertake. Women can die en route, or shortly upon arrival at health facilities. And despite appropriate management upon arrival, women will die. But clinicians cannot not make recommendations that fix blame on patients and their families. If the recommendation suggests that someone outside the room should do something, then the recommendation will be ineffective.

Review of past peer-review recommendations can reveal patterns and needs for change, for example, the need for improvement in labour monitoring may emerge when cases involving intrapartum fetal death, uterine rupture, and postpartum haemorrhage are all reviewed. They all involve separate cases of poor recognition and management of a long, dysfunctional labour. The group may decide on a refresher workshop in the use of the partograph, a protocol drafted regarding management of prolonged labour, and staffing changes to provide better night-time coverage.

Identification of administrative concerns may arise that identify substandard care, such as inconsistent ambulance coverage for transport to a referral center. Or if a policy of not refusing women in an obstetric emergency if her family is unable to pay immediately is not being adhered to because the woman is initially assessed by a non-clinical person at the point of entry, therefore leading to unnecessary delays occurring due to discussions of the cost of care. These systemic gaps can be identified by clinicians and brought to the administrations attention where improvements can be negotiated.

Also, identifying social patterns that lead to poor outcomes can also be part of the review process. Family resistance in referring a woman to a consulting center for care in the event of a complication may be due to the double-billing-for-one-delivery taking place—billing at the primary care facility and at the referral centre. Staff may decide to (1) conduct antenatal education for families about the realities of paying for care, and what to expect (the so-called but likely impossible *financial preparedness*), (2) request the facility administration to offer discounts to families who need to be referred to the consulting center, (3) and staff may consider approaching the referral center for discounts for families being referred from their facility.

Counting Cases in the Community

In addition to intrapartum care, skilled birth attendants usually attend to many reproductive health needs within their community. They may provide counselling for and dispense family planning methods. They may provide some antenatal care—tetanus toxoid injection, iron and calcium supplements, blood pressure monitoring, proteinuria testing, treatment of pre-existing conditions (e.g. hookworm), and assessment of fetal growth. They may provide postpartum follow-up, the minimum which is common is vaccination of the newborn at six to eight weeks of age. This gives the SBA up to three points of contact with women who are at risk of dying from pregnancy-related complications in the community.

Following women can be difficult due to poor civil infrastructure (limited transportation, no phones, no addresses), women returning to their parents' home for delivery, and migration for political-economic reasons. Women may also seek prenatal care at a primary care facility in their community and for delivery, they travel to the referral center to avoid the double-billing-for-one-delivery mentioned above. However, SBAs have an opportunity to ask what the woman's family's plan for care will be for delivery. And if a woman plans to seek the care of this SBA and follow-up postpartum, then if this woman does not come eventually for delivery, the SBA should ask within the community where and how the woman is. This expectation recognizes the SBA as a primary care provider and instills the sense of responsibility with the SBA for the women in their care. 'Unbooked' women should be offered documentation of their visit to carry with them to their next clinical encounter, and efforts should be made to maintain contact with 'booked' women.

The SBA should also document women lost to follow-up and any attempts made to find them. Also, political events that result in a woman's inability to seek care should be included in the chart, such as curfews, transportation strikes, or state of emergency, as this adds to the larger picture of where and how care is being impacted by the society in which the woman lives.

The WHO recommendations regarding post-partum care suggest an optimal (6 hours, 6 days, 6 weeks and 6 months) schedule of visits (*http://www.who.int/reproductive-health/publications/msm_98_3/postpartum_care_mother_newborn.pdf* , Accessed June 14, 2006). However, the reality is that maternal postpartum follow-up has yet to be recognized as important as antenatal care, and it is yet another frontier to be tackled. Postnatal care is an opportunity for the SBA to follow up with the woman regarding self-care, warning signs, and when to seek help. With a lack of appropriate follow-up of women who do not return for care, women who die from postpartum complications are left uncounted despite their contact with an SBA. If clinicians value postnatal care, there can improved care for women at a time when the majority of maternal deaths occur. Postnatal education can take place antenatally, postnatal care could be free following delivery (i.e. the cost is included in the package of care), provision of home visits within 24 hours of the birth, family member can come get the SBA to direct them to the home of the new mother—if directions to the home is difficult, and family-requested home visits following unattended homebirth, or for retained placenta or perineal repair should include follow-up care within 24 hours.

Participation in Facility-based Maternal Death Reviews and Confidential Enquiries into Maternal Deaths (CEMD)

Facility-based audits and CEMD are multidisciplinary endeavors to investigate maternal deaths from a number of different viewpoints.

Peer-review mentioned above makes up part of the surveillance cycle outlined in Beyond the Numbers [24]. For clinicians participating in regular peer-review, their contribution of quality data can be valuable as documentation will be complete.

Facility-based audits involve multidisciplinary peer-review, review of maternal deaths over time, and reviewing maternal deaths across district or regional facilities. The facility-based audit has the benefit of the involvement of more people at high seniority, and with motivation, can lead to improvements in systemic shortfalls in care, such as need for supplies, equipment, special training, or allocation of resources for protocol development.

The UK established a process of CEMD, and the process has been repeated in South Africa and Malaysia. CEMD attempts to identify all maternal deaths, and collect all the information pertaining to and around the death, and piece together the "story" that lead to the woman's death [25]. In South Africa, maternal deaths were made notifiable events and a process is initiated following the death of a woman. Assessors (an obstetrician and midwife) receive and review cases, create a report, and the report is distributed to all involved in the care of women around the time of pregnancy. The primary and final cause of death is identified. Avoidable factors, missed opportunities, and substandard care are identified. Finally, recommendations are provided. Clinicians receive the report and are expected to take steps within their practice to adopt the recommendations [26].

In a Cochrane review of critical incident audits and feedback as effective interventions in reducing maternal mortality, no suitable studies were found [27]. The authors concluded that the data thus far indicated more benefit than harm, and that maternal death reviews should continue to be held.

CONCLUSION

There is and will continue to be a need for ongoing surveillance of maternal deaths, both to establish the magnitude of the problem and to learn from the deaths of women. The role of the skilled birth attendants spans from registration of a pregnancy-related death to acting as an assessor in a national CEMD. It is the responsibility of the skilled birth attendant to strive to improve the quality of care they provide, the quality of the data they produce, and actively advocate for change leading to the reduction of the number of maternal deaths in their community.

KEY POINTS

- global, regional and most national estimates of maternal mortality ratio should be used to raise awareness of the issue and ideally, not for measuring changes over time or country to country comparisons
- process and service indicators (number of skilled birth attendants, number of basic and comprehensive emergency obstetric facilities, number of caesarean sections, and case fatality rate) are proposed proxy measures for estimating maternal mortality ratio
- however, surveillance at a local, and national level is still important to provide ongoing, systematic collection of data which is analyzed and interpreted—to estimate the magnitude of the problem, and evaluate change
- skilled birth attendants have a vital role in ongoing maternal mortality surveillance

- peer-review, facility-based audits and confidential enquires in maternal deaths improve the standard of clinical care delivered by skilled birth attendants, lead to improvements in data quality, and can lead to improved measurement of local, and national maternal mortality ratio.

APPENDICES

Appendix 1—Definitions

Maternal death – the death of a woman while pregnancy or within 42 days of termination of pregnancy, irrespective of the duration and site of the pregnancy, from any cause related to or aggravated by the pregnancy or its management but not from accidental or incidental causes. This provides the *medical cause of death*.

Pregnancy-related death—Maternal death from unspecified cause occurring during pregnancy, labour and delivery, or the puerperium.

Direct obstetric death—deaths resulting form obstetric complications of the pregnant state (pregnancy, labour, and the puerperium), from interventions, omissions, incorrect treatment, or from a chain of events resulting from any of the above.

Indirect obstetric deaths—deaths resulting from previous existing disease or disease that developed during pregnancy and which was not due to direct obstetric causes, but was aggravated by physiologic effects of pregnancy.

Late maternal death—death of a woman from direct or indirect obstetric causes more than 42 days but less than one year after termination of pregnancy.

The Tenth Revision of the International Classification of Diseases (ICD-10), reprinted[1]

Box-1

Maternal mortality ratio (MMRatio) = no. of maternal deaths in a given time/ 100 000 live births

Maternal mortality rate = no. maternal deaths in a given time / 100 000 women of childbearing age

Lifetime risk = 1-(1-maternal mortality rate) [35]

Maternal mortality in 2000: estimates developed by WHO, UNICEF and UNFPA. Geneva: World Health Organization, 2004.

Appendix 2—Obstetric Service Indicators [28]

1. Amount of EmOC per 500 000 population
   - 4 Basic
   - 1 Comprehensive
2. Geographical distribution
   - Basic EmOC within 2 hours of most women

3. At least 15% of all births in the population take place in either Basic or Comprehensive EmOC facilities
4. At least 100% of all women with obstetric complications are treated in Basic or Comprehensive EmOC facilities.
5. Caesarean section rate is not less than 5% and not more than 15%.
6. Case fatality rate of women with complication is not more than 1%.

REFERENCES

[1]   Maternal mortality in 2000: estimates developed by WHO, UNICEF and UNFPA. Geneva: World Health Organization, 2004.

[2]   AbouZahr, C. Safe motherhood: a brief history of the global movement 1947-2002. *British Medical Bulletin,* 2003 67, 13-25.

[3]   Sundari Ravindran, T; Berer, M. Preventing maternal mortality: evidence, resources, leadership, action. In: Berer, M; Sundari Ravindran, T editors. *Safe Motherhood Initiatives: Critical Issues.* London: Blackwell Science Ltd; 1999;1-7.

[4]   Revised 1990 estimates of maternal mortality. A new approach by WHO and UNICEF. Geneva, Switzerland: World Health Organization; 1996.

[5]   Maternal mortality in 1995: Estimates developed by WHO, UNICEF and WNFPA Geneva, Switzerland: World Health Organization; 2001.

[6]   Turner, L; Cyr, M; Kinch, R; Liston, R; Kramer, M; Fair, M; et al. Under-reporting of maternal mortality in Canada: a question of definition. *Chronic Dis Can,* 2002 23(1), 22-30.

[7]   Deneux-Tharaux, C; Berg, C; Bouvier-Colle, M; Gissler, M; Harper, M; Nannini, A; et al. Underreporting of pregnancy-related mortality in the United States and Europe. *Obstetricsand Gynecology,* 2005 106(4), 684-92.

[8]   Gülmezoglu, M; Say, L; Betrán, A; Villar, J; Piaggio, G. WHO systematic review of maternal mortality and morbidity: methodological issues and challenges. *BMC Medical Research Methodology,* 2004 4, 16.

[9]   WHO, ICM, FIGO. Making pregnancy safer: the critical role of the skilled attendant. A joint statement. Geneva: World Health Organization; 2004.

[10] Curtis, S. Midwives and their role in the reduction of direct obstetric deaths during the late nineteenth century: the Sundsvall Region of Sweden (1860-1890). *Medical History,* 2005 49, 321-350.

[11] Loudon, I. Deaths in childbed from the eighteenth century to 1935. *Medical History,* 1986 30, 1-41.

[12] Sloan, N; Winikoff, B; Fikree, F. An ecological analysis of maternal mortality ratios. *Studies in Family Planning,* 2001 32, 352-355.

[13] Betrán, A; Wojdyla, D; Posner, S; Gulmezoglu, A. National estimates for maternal mortality: an analysis based on the WHO systematic review of maternal mortality and morbidity. *BMC Public Health,* 2005 5(1), 131.

[14] De Brouwere, V; Tonglet, R; Van Lerberghe, W. Strategies for reducing maternal mortality in developing countries: what can we learn from the history of the industrialized West? *Tropical Medicine and International Health,* 1998 3(10), 771-782.

[15] Van Lerberghe, W; De Brouwere, V. Of blind alleys and things that have worked: history's lessons on reducing maternal mortality. In: De Brouwere, V; Van Lerberghe, W editors. *Safe motherhood strategies: a review of the evidence*. Antwerp: ITG Press; 2001; 7-33.

[16] Kaunitz, A; Spence, C; Danielson, T RW R; Grimes, D. Perinatal and maternal mortality in a religious group avoiding obstetric care. *Am J Obstet Gynecol*, 1984 150, 826-31.

[17] McCaw-Binns, A. Safe motherhood in Jamaica: from slavery to self-determination. *Paediatric and Perinatal Epidemiology*, 2005 19, 254-261.

[18] de Bernis, L; Sherratt, D; AbdouZahr, C; Van Lerberghe, W. Skilled attendants for pregnancy, childbirth and postnatal care. *Br Med Bull*, 2003 67, 39-57.

[19] Graham, W; Bell, J; Bullough, C. Can skilled attendance at delivery reduce maternal mortality in developing countries? In: De Brouwere, V; Van Lerberghe, W editors. *Safe Motherhood Strategies: a Review of the Evidence*. Antwerp: ITG Press; 2001; 97-130.

[20] WHO. Reproductive health indicators: Guidelines for their generation, interpretation and analysis for global monitoring. Geneva: World Health Organization, 2006.

[21] Shiffman, J. Generating political will for safe motherhood in Indonesia. *Social Science and Medicine*, 2003 56, 1197-1207.

[22] Graham, W. The global problem of maternal mortality: inequalities and inequities. In: MacLean, A; Neilson, J editors. *Maternal Morbidity and Morbidity*. London: RCOG Press; 2002; 3-20.

[23] World Health Organization partograph in management of labour. World Health Organization Maternal Health and Safe Motherhood Programme. *Lancet*, 1994 344(8916), 193.

[24] Boullough, C; Graham, W. Facility-based maternal deaths review: learning from deaths occurring in health facilities. In: Lewis G editor. *Beyond the numbers: Reviewing maternal deaths and complications to make pregnancy safer*. Geneva: World Health Organization; 2004; 57-76.

[25] Lewis, G. Confidential enquiries into maternal death. In: Lewis, G editor. *Beyond the numbers*. Geneva: World Health Organization; 2004.

[26] Pattinson, RC; Moodley, J. Confidential enquiry in maternal deaths in South Africa. In: MacLean, AB NJ editor. *Maternal morbidity and mortality*. London: RCOG Press; 2002.

[27] Pattinson, RC; Say, L; Makin, JD, MH B. Critical incident audit and feedback to improve perinatal and maternal mortality and morbidity. *The Cochrane Database of Systematic Reviews*: The Cochrane Database of Systematic Reviews, 2005 10.1002/14651858.CD002961.pub2

[28] Ronsmans, C; Campbell, OMR; McDermott, J; Koblinsky, M. Questioning the indicators of need for obstetric care. *Bulletin of the World Health Organization*, 2002 80(4), 317-323.

In: Women's Health in the Majority World: Issues and Initiatives   ISBN1-1-60021-493-2
Eds: L. Elit and J. Chamberlain Froese, pp. 49-64   © 2007 Nova Science Publishers, Inc.

Chapter 4

PREVENTING CERVICAL CANCER WORLDWIDE

Laurie Elit[1]

Department of Obstetrics and Gynecology, McMaster University
Juravinski Cancer Centre,
Hamilton Health Sciences Centre, Hamilton, Ontario, Canada

ABSTRACT

Background

For women, cervical cancer is the second most common cancer worldwide. This is unfortunate given that cervical cancer can be preventable through screening programs. If cervical cancer occurs and is identified early, it can be cured with radical surgery or aggressive chemoradiation.

Objective

To review the strategies available to prevent or manage cervical cancer.

Methods and Results

We will review the global impact of cervical cancer, methods of primary (ie., vaccination) and secondary prevention (ie., cyotology, visual inspection with acetic acid). The important aspects of a screening program will be discussed. Key principals in treatment and management of end stage disease will be reviewed.

---

[1] Contact: Dr. Laurie Elit, Juravinski Cancer Centre, 699 Concession Street, Hamilton, Ontario, Canada. L8V 5C2
email: laurie.elit@hrcc.on.ca

Conclusions

Given that cervical cancer is potentially a preventable disease, global strategies toward assessing vaccines, providing screening programs, making available curative treatment and palliative care must be better implemented.

INTRODUCTION

Cervical cancer is the second most common cancer among women world wide and the leading cause of cancer in women in many developing countries. In fact, the annual number of new cervical cancer cases equals the number of maternal deaths in low resource settings [1]. Women in low resource settings who present with cervical cancer usually come with advanced disease, thus the diagnosis of cervical cancer is usally equated with death. In this chapter we will review the global burden of cervical cancer, opportunities for prevention, and treatment option for preinvasive and invasive disease.

1. GLOBAL BURDEN ON CERVICAL CANCER

Low resource countries account for 80% of the worlds total cervical cancer cases. India alone accounts for 25% of the world's burden. In the low resource countries cervical cancer accounts for 15% of cancers in women and the life time risk of cervical cancer is 2% [2]. Unfortunately, in some countries like sub-Saharan Africa, Latin America and Asia, the life-time risk of cervix cancer is much higher at 6-7% [2].

For each death from cervical cancer, it has been estimated that between 14-20 years of potential life before 70 years of age are lost. Assuming that an average of 17 years of life are lost per death this gives an estimate of more than 3.4 million women-years of life lost before 60 years of age due to cervical cancer worldwide [2].

Describing the distribution of disease between different populations and over time is a good way of developing hypothesis about the cause of cancer and quantifying potential for preventive activities [3]. These include development and implementation of health policy through identification of health problems, decision on priorities for preventive and curative programs and evaluation of outcomes of programs of prevention, early detection, screening and treatment in relation to resource inputs.

As we review the trends in cancer incidence and morality some of the limitations of the data over time and between nations must be noted. In 1990, only 18% of the world's population was covered by registries this included 64% of developed countries and 5% of developing countries [4]. More recently, 42% of the world's population is covered by vital registration systems. Information on cancer incidence is only as reliable as the population-based cancer registry that collects information on these cases. In many parts of the world these registries are not well developed [4].

Table 1. Age Standardized Incidence and Mortality Rates from Cervical Cancer.

Region	Incidence Age Standardized Rate	Mortality Age Standardized Rate
World	16.2	9.0
Developed	10.3	4.0
Developing	19.1	11.2
Eastern Africa	19.1	11.2
Middle Africa	28.0	23.0
Southern Africa	38.2	22.6
Western Africa	29.3	23.8
Carribean	32.0	16.0
Central America	30.6	15.0
South America	28.6	12.9
Northern America	7.7	2.3
Eastern Asia	7.4	3.7
South East Asia	18.7	10.2
South Central Asia	26.2	15.0
Western Asia	5.8	2.9
Central and Eastern Europe	14.5	7.1
Northern Europe	9.0	3.6
Southern Europe	10.7	3.3
Western Europe	10	3.4
Australia New Zealand	7.4	2.0
Melanesia	38.1	21.7
Micronesia	9.4	5.2
Polynesia	28.0	15.0

http:/www-dep.iarc.fr/ata/T2_86403018.txt [5]
GLOBCAN 2002

1a. Trends In Cancer Incidence

In 2002 there were 493,243 incident cases of cervical cancer and 273,505 women died of disease [5]. The incidence ASR for the world was 16.2 with 10.3 for the developed world and 19.1 for the developing world. Cervix cancer is the leading cause of cancer among women in the developing countries of sub-saharan Africa, Central and South America and South-east Asia (Table 1).

The incidence of cervical cancer begins to rise at age 20-29 years and peaks between 55-64 years and then declines. The age standardized incidence rates vary from 20-55/100,000 women from 1993-1997. These high rates are seen in Zimbabwe, Uganda, Guinea, Mali, rural India, Peru, Bolivia and north east Brazil. In some regions the rates have stabilized, in others it has decreased (Shanghai); in many countries it has risen (sub-Saharan Africa, Mali, Uganda). In 2002, incidence rates in excess of 50.0 occurred in East Africa (in Zambia, Zimbabwe), South Africa (in Lesotho, Swaziland), Western Africa (in Guinea), Central America (in Belize), and South America (in Bolivia, Paraguay).

Between 80-90% of confirmed cervical cancer cases occur among women age 35 or older. Incidence rates are highest between 50-60 years. Bearing this in mind, cervical screening strategies must focus on these ages. Any changes seen in the incidence of cervical cancer over time reflect the impact of prevention strategies.

1b. Trends in Cancer Mortality

In 2002, there were 493,243 new cervical cancer cases and 273,505 women died . The ASR mortality rate was 9.0 for the world, 4.0 for the developed world and 11.2 for the developing world. There is reliable information available from about 30 developing countries (Table 1). Again the quality of the mortality data from developing countries is variable [4].

The 5 year age standardized relative survival rates in selected developing countries show rates lower in the developing world as compared to the developed world (with the exception of China and Chiang Mai, Thailand) [4]. The mortality ASR exceeded 40 in the following regions Eastern Africa (in Rwanda, Tanzania, Zambia, Zimbabwe), South Africa (in Lesotho and Swaziland), Western Africa (in Guinea), and the Carribean (in Haiti).

The proportion of localized cervical cancer in developing counties is quite low at less than 20%. Reasons for the late diagnosis of disease include: presentation at time of symptoms (which usually means advanced stage); lack of radical surgery in many developing countries [4]; limited access to radiotherapy services (for example only 12 of 47 continental sub-Saharan countries have radiotherapy services and many do not function for much of the time due to lack of radiation sources, personnel or breakdown [4]).

Mortality can be a proxy for the risk of developing disease or can be used to evaluate the effects of early diagnosis or treatment. Thus, education, prevention and improved access to diagnosis and treatment are an important aspect for cervical cancer control.

1c. Cervix Cancer in the Context of Other Diseases

World wide there are 10.1 million new cancer cases, 6.2 million deaths and 22.4 million people living with cancer in 2000 (Table 2). Lung cancer is the leading cause of cancer with 1.2 million cases and 1.1 million deaths annually. Breast cancer affects 1.05 million women but is the fifth cause of death due to favorable prognosis (mortality: incidence = 0.4). Colon cancer is third leading cause of cancer with 945,000 cases and 492,000 deaths. Stomach cancer is the fourth leading cause of cancer with 876,000 cases and 647,000 deaths [3].

For females, the incidence of breast cancer is 1,050,300 and cervix is 470,600. The annual mortality for breast is 373,000, lung 292,700, stomach 241,400, colorectal 237,600 and cervix is 233,400. The prevalence of breast cancer is 3,860,300 followed by cervix at 1,401,400.

Of the 7.1 million deaths from all causes in women 24-64 years old, 6.1 million (86%) occur in the developing world. AIDS accounts from 14.2%, breast cancer for 8.4% and cervical cancer for 2.2% [2].

Table 2. Female Burden of Cancers in Major Organs
in the developing world Incidence per 100,000 [6].

Registry	China	India	Indonesia	Iran	Pakistan	Phillipines	Thailand	Vietnam
Breast	12.7	22.6	14.8	12.3	56.6	47.7	16.3	13.8
Cervix	1.2	25.3	21.7	7.0	7.3	21.6	20.9	13.1
Colorectal	9.0	3.8	6.3	2.9	5.0	15.8	7.5	6.4
Stomach	14.7	3.5	?	5.9	3.2	6.4	1.5	8.5

1d. Years of Life Lost [2]

Years of Life Lost and disability or Quality adjusted life years lost show the impact of priority setting within health-care systems. Yang has presented an excellent review of this topic. The years of life lost (YLL) from cervical cancer in women 25-64 years is 2.7 million YLL; 2.4 million YLL occur are reported for the developing world and 0.3 million in the developed countries. Of the 7 health conditions Yang studied in women (AIDS, Maternal conditions, Tuberculosis, stomach, lung, breast and cervical cancer), cervix cancer was the leading cause of life lost in Latin America and the Caribbean. The risk of losing life from cervical cancer is higher in developing than developed countries. Age standardized rates are more than 2.5 times greater. In subSaharan Africa and South East Asia, AIDS eclipse the other causes of years of life lost. The leading cause of years of life lost is maternal conditions for South Central Asia and Northern Africa immediately followed by tuberculosis. In subSaharan Africa, Central America, and South Eastern and Central Asia, the leading cause of years of life lost from cancer is cervical cancer. The age standardized rates for years of life lost were 3.95 in subSaharan Africa, 4.10 in South Central Asia and 3.21 in Latin America.

2. EPIDEMIOLOGY [7-18]

2a. Global Perspective on HPV

Munoz [19] determined the geographic variation in HPV type distribution in cervical cancer by pooling the data from an international survey of HPV types in cervical cancer and from a multicenter case-control study co-ordinated by the IARC. Included were 3,607 incident cases of cervical cancer from 25 countries. HPV typing was completed using PCR assays. HPV DNA was detected in 96% of the specimens. A single HPV type was detected in 92.2%. The most frequent HPV types were HPV 16 (57.4%), 18 (16.6%) and 45 (6.8%). The leading HPV types for squamous cancers were 16 (54.38%), 18 (11.3%), and 45 (5.2%) and for adeno or adenosquamous, HPV 16 (41.6%), HPV 18 (37.3%) and 45 (6.0%). Geographically, HPV 16 was the most prominant type in sub-Saharan Africa (47.7%) and Europe/North America (69.7%). HPV 18 was the second most common type with prevalence ranging from Central/South America (12.6%) to south Asia (25.7%). HPV 45 was the third most prevalent type; its prevalence was high in sub-Saharan Africa. HPV 31 has a high prevalence in Central and South America. Prevalence of the various HPV types appeared to vary with age.

HPV 16 and 18 account for 70.7% of the types found in cervical cancer while, the top 7 types (16, 18, 45, 31, 33, 52, and 58) account for 87.4% of the cervical cancer cases worldwide. A vaccine that includes either the leading 2 or 7 types of HPV could significantly impact the global cervical cancer burden. Use of an HPV cocktail for screening and management, Munoz's results suggest that the HC2 cocktail including the leading 13 HPVs would detect as positive 91.6% of the cancers.

3. PRIMARY PREVENTION

Primary prevention of cervical cancer can be obtained through prevention and control of genital HPV infection. Health promotion strategies geared at a change in sexual behavior (abstinence or fewer partners, condom use) targeting all sexually transmitted infections of public health significance should be effective in preventing genital HPV infection. An example is the ABC program found in Uganda (A-abstinence, B-Be faithful, C-wear a condom). The strategy of treating infection, counseling and partner notification not currently not recommended outside of a research or evaluation setting.

Primary prevention could also involve immunization against high risk HPV types.

3a. Vaccination

There have been three randomized trials, which assess the role of HPV vaccine using viral like particle (VLP) technology. In the Kousky paper [20], HPV 16 LI VLP vaccine was used in 2, 392 young women. It was well tolerate with no serious adverse effects. There was 100% efficacy against all new cases of HPV 16 infections. The bivalent vaccine against HPV 16 and 18 described by Harper [21] was shown to prevent persistent infections and associated cervical abnormalities over a 27-month period. The focus of this vaccine will likely be to prevent cervical cancer. The new quadravalent vaccine provides immunity to HPV 6, 11, 16, and 18. Villa [22] showed in 277 young women that there was 90% efficacy (95% CI 71-97, p<0.0001) for preventing infection with HPV 6, 11, 16 and 18 at 36 months of follow-up in the vaccine compared to placebo group. The aim of this later vaccine will be vaccination of teenagers to prevent sexually transmitted disease.

These vaccines are only now coming forward for FDA (Federal Drug Agency) approval. It will be at least a decade before we see a drop in the rates of cervical cancers associated with HPV 16 and 18. The effectiveness will in part depend on population coverage with the vaccine. But it is clear that given the many types of HPV involved in the development of cervical cancer, vaccination may markedly decrease the incidence of disease but vaccination will not eliminate the disease.

3b. How Does Cervical Cancer Develop?

The lifetime risk of HPV infection can reach 80% but only about 5% of infected women develop cervical cancer. An HPV infection may result in mild cervical dysplasia which means that in half of the cases the body's immune system will heal the change but in the other group the disease will persist or progress to severe dysplasia. In most cases with time, severe dysplasia will progress to cervical cancer. Certain cofactors appear to be associated with this process like smoking, age and other co-infections (i.e., Chlamydia) [23-28].

3c. Screening

Cervix cancer is a preventable disease. The primary goal of cervical screening is to prevent cervical cancer. This is achieved by the detection, eradication and follow-up of preinvasive cervical lesions. Population based cervical screening programs in the developed world have shown a clear fall in cervical cancer incidence and a stage shift to earlier stage disease [29]. The most common screening strategy is cervical cytology. More recently other low cost techniques have been evaluated including Visual Inspection with Acetic Acid and Visual Inspection with Lugol's solution. The risk of cervical cancer remains high in many developing countries due to the lack of or inefficiencies of existing screening programs.

3d. What Does Screening Mandate?

The goals of any screening test are to identify the disease at a point in its coarse when it is amenable to curative therapy, while simultaneously minimizing adverse impacts to the patient and to those who may have a false positive screen. A screening test must be safe, practical, affordable and available. An ideal screening test should be performed infrequently and be capable of detecting precursor or early easily treatable lesions with great accuracy. Cervical screening options which have come to attention including: cervical cytology, visual inspection with acetic acid (VIA), visual inspection with Lugol's iodine, and HPV testing.

Table 3. Definitions of abnormal cytology.

Dysplasia	Cervical Intraepithelial Neoplasia	Squamous Intraepithelial Lesion
Atypia	Atypia	ASCUS
HPV Effect	HPV Effect	Low Grade SIL
Mild Dysplasia	CIN 1	
Moderate Dysplasia	CIN 2	High Grade SIL
Severe Dysplasia	CIN 3	
Carcinoma In Situ		

3e. Definitions

There are several accepted systems for classifying preinvasive squamous changes in the cervix: dysplasia (atypia, HPV effect, mild, moderate or severe dysplasia/carcinoma in situ); cervical intraepithelial neoplasia (CIN) (atypia, HPV effect, CIN 1, 2, 3) and Squamous Intraepithelial Lesion (SIL) or the Bethesda System (Atypical squamous cells of undetermined significance (ASCUS); low grade and high grade SIL) (Table 3). All these systems recognize increasing levels of atypical cellular appearance. In this manuscript we will refer to the Bethesda system for cytology and the CIN system for histology.

3f. Cervical Cytology

Aureli Babes in Presse Medicale first described cervical cytology on 11April 1928. The original paper by Papanicolaou and Traut described the concept of mass screening for precursors of carcinoma of the uterine cervix in 1943. The sampling of the cervix by means of a scraper (ie. the Ayre's spatula) was never tested in a double-blind study. There have been no randomized controlled trials of cytology screening efficacy to demonstrate cervical cancer morbidity or mortality reduction because the Pap test became established in an era when evidence of medical benefit relied on lesser standards of proof. After 4 decades in which the Pap test occupied a niche in the medical armamentarium it is not possible to supplement that of observational epidemiology. What is clear is that when cervical cytologic screening was used widely, cervical cancer rates fell. In Iceland, a national program for cervical cancer screening was launched in 1960 and reaches almost all women in the country. There has been an 80% decrease in the rates of cervical cancer deaths over a 20-year period . In contrast, only an estimated 5% of women in developing countries have had Pap smears in the last five years This test became employed widely as it detected abnormal cells that were not visible to the naked eye. It has taken several decades to understand the limitation of this test.

The major problem with cervical cytology is the high false negative result (low sensitivity). About two-thirds of false negatives are due to poor sample collection and slide preparation and one-third of cases are attributable to slide interpretation errors. Thin prep and automated technologies are attempts to improve performance by making slides easier to read. Specificity is also a problem and the Bethesda system of cytological diagnoses was an attempt to provide uniformity in terminology. It has failed though in categorizing borderline or equivocal smears. The result has been an increase in number of repeat cytologies or colposcopies with an increased financial burden to the health care system. In addition the cervical cytology approach fails if it is based on opportunistic screening rather than population based, long intervals between smears, low-quality cytology assessment, inadequate management guidelines and lack of follow-up. In contrast, programs with good quality control have likely met their ceiling in terms of cervical cytology sensitivity.

Although cervical cytology is a reasonable screening test for cervical cancer, cytology-screening programs are difficult to organize, require a sophisticated infrastructure (i.e., highly trained personal, adequately equipped laboratories, referral systems to communicate results), and may not be feasible for many developing countries with other competing public health priorities such as clean drinking water. Thus lower cost methods of diagnosing preinvasive disease have been explored.

3g. VIA – Visual Inscpection with Acetic Acid [30]

VIA involves applying a dilute vinegar solution (3-5% acetic acid) to the cervix. It dehydrates the cells and causes surface coagulation of cellular proteins thereby reducing the transparency of the dysplastic epithelium. These changes are more pronounced in abnormal epithelium where nuclear density and protein concentration are high. This change can be detected with the naked eye and constitutes a positive VIA test. The advantages of VIA are that it is easy to learn, it does not require a lab infrastructure, the results are immediate and may allow for immediate colposcopy/biopsy or treatment, and the cost of supplies is low. Personnel costs depend on the qualifications of the staff performing the test and the staff cost in a country.

There have been several cross-sectional studies conducted in China, India, Zimbabwe and South Africa that show sensitivity similar to that of cytology for detecting high-grade cervical disease and invasive cancer but lower specificity. The average sensitivity is 76.5% and the average specificity is 80.2%. for cytology the sensitivity is 75% and specificity is 90.7%. This means that with VIA more patients will be referred for colposcopy or immediate treatment that in the cytology assessed group.

3h. VILI – Visual Inspection with Lugol's Iodine

VILI involves painting the cervix with Lugol's Iodine which stains glycogenated cells and does not stain endocervical cells, denuded epithelium or dysplastic cells. VIA has a superior sensitivity and specificity compared to VILI.

3j. HPV Testing

A single lifetime screen for oncogenic HPV in the woman over 30 years old is another screening strategy being explored in the developing world. Whether this is a health care professional collected sample or a self-collected sample is currently being explored. Cuzick [31] has review the randomized trials on primary screening using HPV testing (Table 4).

Table 4. Studies describing HPV testing as a primary screening strategy

Location	Size	Age	Strategy	Sensitivity	Specificity
England Hart [31]	11,085	30-60yr	Cytology HPV II Outcome >/= CIN 2	76.6% 97.1%	95.8% 93.3%
Hammersmith	2988	> 35 yr	Cytology HPV II	Study is ongoing	
German	8,967	> 30 yr	Cytology HPV	Study is ongoing	
Jena	5455	18-70 yr	Cytology HPV II and Colp	Study is ongoing	
French	14,122	15-76 yr	Cytology HPV II	Study is ongoing	
Holland Bulkmans [32]	21,966	29-61 yr	HPV Outcome >/=CIN 3	Study is ongoing	

Oncogenic HPV positive was 97.1% sensitive for histology showing CIN 2 or worse compared to 76.7% for cytology. The specificity of HPV for negative histology was 93.3% compared to cytology which was 95.8%. The sensitivity of oncogenic HPV positivity for low-grade lesions was 65% compared to cytology of 30%. Cuzick suggests that HPV testing could be used for primary screening in women older than 30 years with cytology as triage of HPV positive women. This strategy would improve detection of CIN 2 or worse without increasing referrals to colposcopy.

Some of the explanations for poor coverage of cervical cytologic screening include the inconvenience, time and discomfort associated with obtaining Pap smears. The technique for acquiring the HPV sample can be by a health care provider obtaining a cervical sample directly or by self-sampling from the vagina [33]. Ogilvie's [34] meta-analysis shows that the sensitivity of Dacron cotton swabs or cytobrushes is 0.74 (95%CI 0.61- 0.84) and specificity 0.88 (95%CI 0.83-0.92). Use of tampon collection method showed sensitivity between 0.67-0.94 and specificity of 0.80-0.85. This specimen collection approach could be used to those women reluctant or unwilling to undergo a pelvic examination because of cultural or personal concerns, or in areas of geographic isolation. If the woman is aware of the limitations of self-collection as compared to clinician collected specimen but would otherwise not have a Pap test, then self-collection may be an option.

3l. Other Screening Tests of Low Interest

Unaided Visual Inspection

Using a naked-eye speculum exam with a good light is referred to as an unaided visual inspection of the cervix. The goal is to identify a cervical cancer at an earlier stage. Trials assessing the value of this test have mainly been carried out in India. The criteria for an abnormal cervix can vary (discharge, growth, ulcer) or (bleeding on touch, bleeding erosions, hypertrophied, elongated, edematous, growth, ulcer). The sensitivity and specificity of finding cancer are both in excess of 90%. The sensitivity and specificity of detecting CIN 3 ranges from 38%-96% .

3k. Cost-Effectiveness of Cervical Cancer Screening in Developing Countries

Susan Goldie used a computer-based model to assess the cost-effectiveness of a variety of cervical cancer screening strategies in 5 countries – India, Kenya, Peru, South Africa and Thailand. She showed that the most cost-effective strategies were those that required the fewest visits. Once in a lifetime screening at the age of 35 years with a one or two-visit strategy involving VIA or DNA testing for HPV reduced the lifetime risk of cancer by 25-36% and cost less than $500 per life year saved. If there were 2 screens at 35 and 40 years, there was an additional 40% decline in cancer. The cost was less than each country's per capita gross domestic product per year of life saved. Thus one clinic visit VIA or DNA testing for HPV is a cost-effective alternative to three-visit cytology based screening programs in resource-poor settings.

There is one paper addressing the incorporation of vaccine use into cervical screening. They showed that vaccination plus biennial screening delayed until age 24 years has the most attractive cost-effectiveness ratio compared to screening only beginning at age 18 years and conducted every 3 years [35]. A strategy of vaccination with annual screening beginning at age 18 has the largest overall reduction in cancer incidence and mortality. The cost-effectiveness of vaccination plus delayed screening is very dependent on age of vaccination, duration of vaccine efficacy and cost of the vaccine.

Conclusion on Screening

Any screening test will compete for funding with other pressing health problems (i.e., communicable diseases). The lessons that have been learned through cytologic screening is that transient low-grade lesions are primarily seen in younger women thus delaying screening until mid-30s is a more efficient strategy for reducing cancer mortality. Screening is less effective against rapidly progressing cancers with proportionately smaller reductions in cancer incidence in younger women compared to women in their 40-50s. The cost of vaccination can be in part achieved by delaying the onset of screening.

4. TREATMENT

4a. See and Treat: Immediate Treatment with Cryotherapy

In much of the developing world access to tests like colposcopy is severely limited. Thus an approach of seeing a patient with an abnormal cytology or VIA result is followed by immediate treatment. Cryotherapy involves holding a low-temperature probe against the cervix to freeze abnormal cells. The equipment has a low cost and training is relatively simple. Cryotherapy is 95% effective in treating severe abnormalities. Cryotherapy failures usually occur if the lesion is larger than the cryotherapy probe or adequate freezing does not take place.

4b. Colposcopy and Treatment Following Biopsy

Hinselmann introduced colposcopy in 1925. Colposcopy became used more consistently in the late 1960's.

Colposcopy in the developed world is used to further evaluate the woman with an abnormal cytologic smear. Using 5-30 fold magnification, 3-5% acetic acid, Lugol's-s solution and green filters, and the cervix can be assessed for the nature and extent of an abnormal epithelial lesion. An abnormal lesion is usually verified histologically. The meta-analysis by Mitchell [36] shows that the average weighted sensitivity of colposcopy for the threshold normal compared with all cervix abnormalities (atypia, CIN 1-3 and cancer) was 96% and the average weighted specificity is 48%. For the threshold normal cervix and CIN 1 compared to CIN 2, 3 and cancer, the average weighted sensitivity was 85% and average weighted specificity 69%. Area under the ROC curve were 0.80 for the threshold normal cervix compared with all abnormalities and 0.82 for the threshold normal cervix and CIN 1 compared with CIN 2,3 and cancer. The low specificity is related to overcalling low-grade lesions.

Histological confirmation of a persistent low-grade lesion or documentation of a high grade lesion is followed by treatment. Studies have shown that all methods: Laser evaporation, laser excision, loop electrosurgical excision procedure (LEEP), cold knife cone and double freeze cryotherapy have excellent and equivocal efficacy. They differ in the amount of cervical stromal damage and the percent of satisfactory squamocolumnar junction in follow-up.

5. FOLLOW-UP

Whichever management strategy is used, the woman will require follow-up. Approximately 10% of women will have a persistent abnormality despite treatment and will require retreatment.

6. TREATMENT OF INVASIVE CERVICAL CANCER

For invasive disease less that 3 mm deep, cone biopsy with negative margins or simple hysterectomy is acceptable [37]. For disease less that 4 cm diameter involving only the cervix, either radical hysterectomy and pelvic node dissection or radical external field radiation with intracavitary boost is recommended [37]. For most advanced disease, chemoradiation with cisplatin chemotherapy provides optimal results. In the event that that a patient cannot be cured, palliative care including adequate pain management and control of symptoms (ie., bleeding, dischange) need to be available.

7. CERVICAL CANCER CONTROL STRATEGY [38]

A cervical cancer control strategy aims to prevent cancer, cure cancer and to increase survival and quality of life for those who develop cancer by converting the knowledge gained through research, surveillance or outcome evaluation into strategies and actions. The continuum of cancer includes prevention, screening, diagnosis, treatment, supportive care/rehabilitation and palliative care. The Grand Challenge is for federal governments and research agencies to invest in developing, implementing and evaluating a cancer control strategy.

Education: Prevention aims a reducing exposure to risk factors and to increase exposure to protective factors. For cervical diseases this includes education of young women and their parents about risk factors and abstinence. It will soon include education around the benefits of vaccination.

Screening: Screening is the early detection of cancer, precursors of cancer or susceptibility to cancer in individuals who do not have symptoms of cancer. These interventions are directed to entire populations or to large and easily identifiable groups within the population. For cervical cancer this would include educating health care workers which could be physicians but could also be trained midwives and nurses in carrying out a strategies such as cervical cytology, VIA, of HPV testing.

Communication: Diagnosis involves timely assessment of symptoms, effective use of investigations, accurate reporting and communication back to the patient.

Treatment of a patient with a confirmed diagnosis may mean LEEP or cone for preinvasive disease or radical surgery for early cervical cancer or chemoradiation for advanced disease.

Supportive care/Rehabilitation is the provision of the necessary services as defined by those living with or affected by cancer to meet their needs (physical, social, emotional, nutritional, informational, psychological, spiritual and practical).

Palliative Care in 2000 means that no-one with cancer needs to die in uncontrolled pain. Reality is not the ideal. Palliative care is the active total care of patients whose disease is beyond curative treatment. The control of pain, symptoms or other problems is important. The goal of palliative care is the best quality of life for patients and their families.

Surveillance is the tracking and forecasting of health determinant through the collection of data and its integration, analysis and interpretation. A well-developed informatics system should include documentation of cancer cases, their treatment and their outcome. This system should also contain screening results, treatment and follow-up information. It is important for this registry to recall patients with abnormal results and have this information available to the health care staff at the time of the patient assessment.

Human resource planning means the identification of personnel needs and training appropriate individuals. For example in cervix cancer there is a need for colposcopists, radical surgeons, radiation oncologists and therapists.

A comprehensive cervical control strategy will address all of these issues.

8. CONCLUSION

Cervical cancer is the second leading cause of cancer among women in the world. Cervical cancer arises from infection with oncogenic HPV. Cervical cancer is preventable through either vaccination or screening strategies. Implementing these strategies well across all economic stratum is necessary in order to reduce and possibly eliminate this disease.

KEY POINTS

- Cervical cancer is the second most common cause of cancer in the world.
- Cervix cancer arises from infection with oncogenic HPV. The most common types are 16,17,45 and 56.
- Vaccination has been proven effective in preventing infection with the HPV type used in the vaccine and preinvasive disease associated with that HPV type.
- Screening can markedly decrease the rates of cervical cancer. Screening tests include: cervical cytology, VIA and HPV testing.

REFERENCES

[1]   Royal Thai College of Obstetrician and Gynecologists (RTCOG), JHPIEGO. Safety, acceptability and feasibility of a single-visit approach to cervical-cancer prevention in rural Thailand: a demonstration project. *Lancet,* 2003 361, 814-820.

[2]   Yang, BH; Bray, FI; Parkin, DM; Sellors, J; Zhang, Z. Cervical cancer as a priority for prevention in different world regions: an evaluation using years of life lost. *Int J Cancer,* 2004 109, 418-424.

[3]   Parkin, DM; Bray, F; Ferlay, J; Pisani, P. Estimating the World Cancer Burden: Globocan 2000. *Int J Cancer,* 2001 94,153-156.

[4]   Sankaranarayanaan, R. Cervical cancer in developing countries. *Transactions of the Royal Society of Tropical Medicine and Hygiene,* 2002 96, 580-585.

[5]   GLOBCAN 2002. IARC. GLOBCAN; 2002; *http:/www-dep.iarc.fr/ata/T2_864030 18.txt.*

[6]   Moore, MA; Tajima, K; Anh, PH; Aydemir, G; Basu, PS; et al. Grand Challenges in Global Health and the Practical Prevention Program? Asian Focus on Cancer Prevention in Femails of the developing world. *Asian Pacific Journal of Cancer Prevention,* 2003 4,153-165.

[7]   Ziegler, RG; Brinton, L; Hamman, RF; Lehman, HF; Levine, RS; Mallin, K. Diet and the risk of invasive cancer among white women in the United States. *Am J Epidemiol,* 1990 132, 432-445.

[8]   Campion, MJ; Berek, J; Hacker, NF editors. *Practical Gynecologic Oncology. Preinvasive Disease.* Philadelphia, PA: Lippincott Williams and Wilkins; 2005; p. 265-336.

[9]   Franco, EL; Villa, LL; Richardson, H; et al. New developments in cervical cancer screening and prevention. In: Franco, E; Monsonego, J editors. *Epidemiology of cervical human papillomavirus infection.* Oxford: Blackwell Science; 1997; 14-22.

[10]   Bosch, FX; Sanjose, S; Castellsague, X; et al. Anonymous 2005; *Geographical and Social Patterns of Cervical Cancer Incidence.*

[11]   Lorincz, AT; Temple, GF; Kurman, RJ; Jensen; AB; Lancaster, WD. Oncogenic association of specific human papillomavirus tpes with cervical neoplasia. *J Natl Cancer Inst,* 1987 79, 671-677.

[12]   Munoz, MM; Bosch, FX; Shah, V; et al. The epidemiology of cervical cancer and human papillomavirus. In: Munoz, MM; Bosch, FX; Shah, V; Meheus, A editors. *The epidemiology of cervical cancer and human papillomavirus.* Lyon, France: IARC; 1992.

[13]   Schiffman, MH; Bauer, HM; Hoover, RN; Glass, AG; Cadell, DM;Rush, BB. Epidemiologic evidence showing that human papillomavirus causes most cervical intraepithelial neoplasia. *J Natl Cancer Inst,* 1993 85, 958-964

[14]   zur Hausen, H. Immortalisation of human cells and their malignant conversion by high risk human papillomavirus genotypes. *Semin Cancer Biol,* 1999, 405-411.

[15]   Bosch, FX; Rohan, T; Schneider, A; Frazer, I; Pfister, H;Castellsague, X. Papillomavirus research update: highlights of the Barcelona HPV 2000 international papillomavirus conference. *J Clin Pathol,* 2001 54,163-175.

[16] Broker, TR. Structure and genetic expression of human papillomaviruses. *Obstet Gynecol Clin North Am,* 1987 14, 329-348.

[17] Hawthorn, RJ; Murdoch, JB; McLean, AB; McKie, RM. Langerhan's cells and subtypes of human papillomavirus in cervical intraepithelial neoplasia. *BMJ,* 1988 297, 643-646.

[18] Schafer, A; Friedmann, W; Mielke, M; Schwartlander, B; Bell, JA. The increased frequency of cervical dysplasia-neoplasia in women infected with the human immunodeficiency virus is related to the degree of immunosuppression. *Am J Obstet Gynecol,* 1991 164, 593-599.

[19] Munoz, N; Bosch, FX; Castellsague, X; Diaz, M; de Sanjose, S; Hammouda, D. Against which human papillomavirus types shall we vaccinate and screen? The international perspective. *Int J Cancer,* 2004 111, 278-285.

[20] Koutsky, L; Ault, KA; Wheeler, CM. A controlled trial of a human papillomavirus type 16 vaccine. *NEJM, 2002* 347,1645-1651.

[21] Harper, DM; Franco, EL; Wheeler, CM. Efficacy of a bivalent L1 virus-like particle vaccine in prevention of infection of human papillomavirus type 16 and 18 in young women: a randomised controlled trial. *Lancet, 2004* 364,1757-1765.

[22] Villa, LL; Costa, RLR; Petta, CA; Andrade, RP; Ault, KA; Giuliano, AR. Prophylactic quadrivalent human papillomavirus (types 6,11,16 and 18) L1 virus-like particle vaccine in young women: a randomised double-blind placebo-controlled multicentre phase II efficacy trial. *Lancet Oncology,* 2005 6, 271-278.

[23] Schiffman, M; Haley, NJ; Fenton, JS; Andrews, AW; Kaslow, RA;Lancaster, WD. Biochemical epidemiology of cervical neoplasia: measuring cigarette smoke constituents in the cervix. *Cancer Res,* 1987 47, 3886-3888.

[24] Ferenczy, A; Coutlee, F; Franco, EL; Hankins, CA. Human papillomavirus and HPV coinfection and the risk of neoplasias of the lower genital tract: a review of recent developments. *CMAJ,* 2003 169, 431-434.

[25] Clark, EA; Hatcher, J; McKeown-Eyssen, GE; Lickrish, GM. Cervical dysplasia: association with sexual behavior, smoking and oral contraceptive use? *Am J Obstet Gynecol,* 1985 151, 612-616.

[26] Syrajanen, K; Varyrynen, M; Casren, O; Yliskoski, M; Mantijarvi, R; Pyrhonen, S. Sexual behavior of women with human papillomavirus (HPV) lesions of the uterine cervix. *Br J Vener Dis,* 1984 60, 243-248.

[27] Ye, Z; Thomas, DB; Ray, RM. Combined oral contraceptive and risk of cervical carcinoma in situ: WHO collaborative study of neoplasia and steroid contraceptives. *Int J Epidmiol,* 1995 24.

[28] Bosch, FX; Munoz, N; Castellsague, X; et al. Male Role in Cervical Carcinogenesis: Lessons from the Studies in Colombia and Spain and a Challenge for the Future. In: Franco, E; Monsonego, J editors. *New Developments in Cervical Cancer Screening and Prevention.* Victoria, Australia: Blackwell Science; 1997; 34-7.

[29] Laara E; Day, NE; Hakama, Matti. "Trends in Mortality From Cervical Cancer in the Nordic Countries: Association with Organized Screening Programmes," *Lancet* 1987;1(8544):1247-9.

[30] Sankaranarayanan, R; Syamalakumari, B; Wesley, R; et al. Visual Inspection as a Screening test for cervical cancer control in developing countries. In: Franco, E; Monsonego, J; editors. *New Developments in cervical cancer screening and prevention.* Victoria, Australia: Blackwell Science; 1997; 411-23.

[31] Cuzick, J; Szarewski, A; Cubie, H; Hulman, G; Kitchener, H;Luesley, D. Management
      of women who test positive for high-risk types of human papillomavirus: the HART
      study. *Lancet,* 2003 362,1871-1876.
[32] Bulkmans, NWJ; Rozendaal, L; Snuders, PJF; Voorhorst, FJ; Boeke, AJP; Zandwuken,
      GRJ. POBASCAM, a Population-based randomized controlled trial for implementation
      of high-risk HPV testing in cervical screening design, methods and baseline data of
      44,102 women. *Int J Cancer,* 2004 110, 94-101.
[33] Becker, D; Siebert, U; Thaler, CJ; Keimeir, D; Hepp, H; Hillemanns, P. Primary
      cervical cancer screening by self-sampling of human papillomavirus DNA in internal
      medicine outpatient clinics. *Ann Oncol,* 2004 15, 863-869.
[34] Ogilvie, GS; Patrick, DM; Schulzer, M; Sellors, JW; Petric, M; Chambers, K; White, R;
      FitzGerald, JM. Diagnostic accuracy of self collected vaginal specimens for human
      papillomavirus compared to clinician collected human papillomavirus specimens: a
      meta-analysis. *Sex Transm Dis,* 2005 81, 207-212.
[35] Kulasingam, SL; Myers, ER. Potential Health and economic impact of adding a human
      papillomavirus vaccine to screening programs. *JAMA,* 2005 290, 781-789.
[36] Mitchell, MF; Schottenfeld, D; Tortolero-Luna, G; Cantor, SB; Richards-Kortum, R.
      Colposcopy for the diagnosis of squamous intraepithelial lesions: a meta-analysis.
      Obstet Gynecol, 1998 91, 626-631.
[37] Staging classification and clinical practice guidelines FIGO 2006
[38] *Alliance for Cervical Cancer Prevention. Preventing Cervical Cancer* .Worldwide.
      2004; 1-24

In: Women's Health in the Majority World: Issues and Initiatives   ISBN1-1-60021-493-2
Eds: L. Elit and J. Chamberlain Froese, pp. 65-107   © 2007 Nova Science Publishers, Inc.

Chapter 5

ANEMIA - CAN ITS WIDESPREAD PREVALENCE AMONG WOMEN IN DEVELOPING COUNTRIES BE IMPACTED? A CASE STUDY: EFFECTIVENESS OF A LARGE-SCALE, INTEGRATED, MULTIPLE-INTERVENTION NUTRITION PROGRAM ON DECREASING ANEMIA IN GHANAIAN AND MALAWIAN WOMEN

Carolyn MacDonald[1], Alison Mildon[1], Mike Neequaye[2], Rose Namarika[3] and Miriam Yiannakis[3]

[1] Nutrition, World Vision Canada;
[2] World Vision Ghana;
[3] World Vision Malawi

ABSTRACT

Objective

To understand the widespread prevalence of anemia in the developing world and its devastating impact on women and children.

Methods

This chapter addresses the prevalence, etiology and consequences of anemia. Treatment options are review. Programs which have been effective in reducing anemia like the MICAH program are discussed in detail. This program is based on the principals

---

[1] Email: *Carolyn_macdonald@worldvision.ca*, Phone: 905 565-6200 ext 3396, Fax: 905 696-2164

of evidence, comprehensive multipronged interventions, and collaborative partnerships with the government, health system and community.

Conclusion

Anemia has devastating consequences for women and children, but comprehensive programs have been shown to decrease the devastation of this disease.

1.0. ANEMIA IN WOMEN: A GLOBAL HEALTH PRIORITY

1.1. Introduction

Anemia, defined as blood hemoglobin level below established cut-off points, is a pervasive global public health problem. An estimated 2 billion people are affected, or more than one third of the world's population [1]. Anemia prevalence is highest in developing countries. Although both males and females of all ages are affected, the most vulnerable groups are pregnant women and young children. Worldwide, more than 50% of pregnant women and over 30% of all women suffer from anemia.[2]

The devastating consequences of anemia in women range from increased fatigue, decreased cognitive ability, decreased work productivity and consequent economic costs of increased morbidity and mortality. In fact, women with severe anemia in pregnancy have a 3.5 times greater chance of dying from obstetric complications compared with non-anemic pregnant women.[3]

Iron deficiency is the most prevalent nutritional deficiency and the major cause of anemia worldwide. The World Health Organization (WHO) estimates that iron deficiency is responsible for approximately 50% of all anemia cases[4] Other significant causes, the relative contributions of which vary by geographic location, include deficiencies of other nutrients, malaria, helminth (worm) infections, and a variety of other diseases. Effective management of anemia in high prevalence contexts requires an analysis of the main contributors, and implementation of an integrated package of interventions to address all major causes.

The international community, through the United Nations, has committed to reducing the global prevalence of anemia by one third by 2010.[5] This presents an enormous challenge, as progress towards achievement of similar previously established goals has been very limited.[6] Despite the high prevalence and serious consequences of anemia, there have been few reported studies assessing the effectiveness of anemia prevention and control programs in developing countries. Moreover, although it is well known that anemia is a result of multiple causes, there are few reported examples of integrated programs addressing the various causes, or assessments of the effectiveness of combining several interventions on anemia prevalence among women. This chapter examines these issues in further detail and presents a case study of a comprehensive nutrition and health program, demonstrating that with effective programming, the international target for the reduction of anemia prevalence in women can be achieved.

1.2. Prevalence of Anemia in Women

1.2.1. Definition of Anemia

Anemia is defined as a low level of hemoglobin in the blood, resulting in lower quantities of oxygen available to support the body's activities. Internationally accepted hemoglobin values which define anemia in women are shown in table 1. These values are applicable to most populations but need to be adjusted for high-altitude locations.

Table 1. Blood Hemoglobin Values (g/dL) Defining Anemia in Women[7]*.

	All Anemia	Mild Anemia	Moderate Anemia	Severe Anemia
Pregnant women	<11.0	10.0-10.9	7.0-9.9	<7.0
Non-pregnant women of childbearing age (>15 years)	<12.0	10.0-11.9	7.0-9.9	<7.0

* WHO/UNICEF/UNU. Iron deficiency anaemia: assessment, prevention, and control. Geneva: World Health Organization; 2001. (WHO/NHD/01.3).

1.2.2. Prevalence of Anemia

At the national level, anemia is considered a severe public health problem when the prevalence is equal to or greater than 40 percent in a vulnerable group (table 2). Based on this criteria, anemia is a severe public health program in nearly all developing countries, as illustrated by the data presented in tables 3-5. On the other hand, anemia prevalence in most industrialized countries is typically in the range of normal to mild public health significance.

Table 2. Public Health Significance of Anemia [8].

Anemia Prevalence	Public Health Significance
≥40%	Severe
20-39%	Moderate
5-19%	Mild
0-4.9%	Normal

Tables 3 and 4 show estimates of anemia prevalence for developing countries and different world regions. For all age groups, the risk of developing anemia is two to seven times greater in developing countries than in industrialized countries, and anemia prevalence is higher in rural areas compared with urban areas.[9]

**Table 3. Prevalence of Anemia in Women,
Developing and Industrialized Countries, 1998 [10].**

	Non-pregnant Women (%)	*Pregnant Women (%)*
Developing Countries	43	55
Industrialized Countries	11	19

Table 4. Anemia Prevalence Rates in Women, Selected Countries (by WHO region).

WHO Region Country, Year	Pregnant Women				Breastfeeding Women				Non-pregnant/Non-breastfeeding				All Women (15-49 yrs)			
	Total %	Severe %	Moderate %	Mild %	Total %	Severe %	Mode-rate %	Mild %	Total %	Severe %	Mode-rate %	Mild %	Total %	Severe %	Mode-rate %	Mild %
Africa																
Cameroon, 2004	51	0.7	31	19	43	0.4	10	33	44	1.0	9	34	46	0.9	12	33
Ghana, 2003	65	1.2	27	37	49	0.9	8	40	42	0.9	8	33	45	0.8	9	35
Tanzania, 2004	59	2.7	33	23	48	0.7	11	36	47	1.2	13	33	49	1.2	15	33
Uganda, 2000/1	41	2.0	17	22	32	0.4	6	26	27	0.6	6	20	31	0.7	8	22
Americas																
Bolivia, 2003	38	0.5	19	18	43	0.8	8	34	30	0.3	5	25	33	0.4	7	26
Haiti, 2000	64	3.7	30	30	52	2.2	14	36	55	3.2	15	37	55	3.0	16	36
Peru, 2000	39	2.0	17	20	40	0.2	7	33	29	0.2	5	24	31	0.3	6	25
South Eastern Asia																
India (1998/99)	50	2.5	25	22	57	1.6	16	39	50	1.9	13	35	52	1.9	15	35
Nepal (1997/98)	75	5.7	68.9	68.9	-	-	-	-	67	1.7	65	65	-	-	-	-
Eastern Mediterranean																
Egypt, 2000	46	0.6	10	35	31	0.2	4	27	26	0.3	4	22	29	0.3	5	24
Jordan, 2002	37	0.1	13	24	28	0.0	4	24	28	0.2	6	22	29	0.1	7	22
Europe																
Turkmenistan, 2000	-	-	-	-	-	-	-	-	-	-	-	-	47	1.1	8	38
Western Pacific																
Cambodia, 2000	66	4.3	35	27	67	2.6	17	47	56	0.7	10	45	58	1.3	13	44

Source: Demographic and Health Surveys, Macro International and the governments of the countries.

Anemia prevalence is highest in the South East Asia, Eastern Mediterranean and Africa regions, with the highest rates found in pregnant women (Table 5).

Table 5. Anemia Prevalence in Pregnant Women, 1998[11].

WHO Region	Anemia Prevalence (%)
Africa	51
Americas	35
E. Mediterranean	55
Europe	25
South East Asia[*]	75
Western Pacific	43
[*] includes South Asia	

The fact that anemia prevalence in many areas persists at moderate to severe levels according to internationally accepted standards primarily reflects the difficulty of meeting the dietary iron needs of women. However there are several other key causes of anemia, which vary in their significance by geographic region. Understanding the main causes of anemia and interventions to address them is a critical component of any effort that aims to reduce the global burden of anemia in women.

1.3. Causes of Anemia and Interventions to Address Them

Hemoglobin is a component of red blood cells, responsible for transporting oxygen to the body's tissues. Anemia results when hemoglobin concentration falls below accepted levels, due to either compromised production, excessive destruction or excessive loss of red blood cells. The major factors directly causing these alterations in red blood cell levels are shown in Table 6.

Table 6. Major Causes of Anemia.

Compromised Red Blood Cell Production	Excessive Red Blood Cell Destruction	Excessive Red Blood Cell Loss
poor dietary iron intake and/or absorption (causes 50% of anemia) poor dietary intake and/or absorption of vitamins A, B12, folate HIV/AIDS infectious disease (e.g., chronic diarrhea; TB) Genetic blood disorders (e.g., sickle cell trait, thalassemia)	malaria	helminth infections (e.g. hookworm, schistosomiasis) bacterial or viral infections reproduction contraception (IUD)

On a global scale, the major causes of anemia in decreasing order of significance are iron deficiency; other nutritional deficiencies; malaria; helminth infections; chronic infections such as HIV/AIDS; reproductive causes; and genetic conditions.[12] These are discussed in further detail below, along with the interventions that can be used to address them.

1.3.1. Iron Deficiency

The mineral iron has many functions in the body. One of these is its role as a component of hemoglobin, the oxygen-transporting molecule in red blood cells. However, iron deficiency is widespread and as the single greatest cause of anemia, is responsible for more than half the global cases of anemia.[13] Lack of adequate dietary iron intake is central to the development of iron deficiency and is a major nutritional issue in developing countries. In addition, iron deficiency is exacerbated through excessive blood loss as a result of infections, menstruation, childbirth and the post partum period.

Iron is the only nutrient for which women have higher requirements than men, due to the regular blood losses experienced during menstruation. Pregnancy, a period of rapid growth and expansion of blood volume, further increases women's need for iron. Iron requirements for different age/sex groups are shown in Box 1. Given the need for a high iron intake to compensate for menstrual losses and the demands of pregnancy, it is not surprising that women are particularly vulnerable to iron deficiency and anemia.

Box 1. Daily Iron Requirements (mg) for Selected Age Groups in Relation to Dietary Iron Bioavailability[14].

Age Group	Sex	Iron Bioavailability of the Diet:[*]		
		High	Medium	Low
1-3 years	both	3.9	5.8	11.6
4-6 years	both	4.2	6.3	12.6
7-10 years	both	5.9	8.9	17.8
11-14 years	M	9.7	14.6	29.2
	F	21.8	32.7	65.4
15-17 years	M	12.5	18.8	37.6
	F	20.7	31	62
18+ years	M	9.1	13.7	27.4
	F[**]	19.6	29.4	58.8
Lactating women		10	15	30

[*]See Box 2 for an explanation of diets of varying levels of iron bioavailability
[**]Non-pregnant, non-lactating, pre-menopausal

In contrast with the high iron needs of women, typical diets in many countries provide very little iron or iron that is poorly absorbed by the body. Both the quantity and quality of dietary iron intake contribute to iron status. The iron sources with greatest bioavailability (i.e. most readily absorbed and utilized by the body) are from animal products, which contain heme iron. Plant sources of iron (such as grains, legumes, vegetables and nuts) are non-heme, and are much more poorly absorbed. See Box 2 for examples of diets with varying levels of iron bioavailability.

Box 2. Characteristics of Diets with Varying Iron Bioavailability[15].

Low Bioavailability	Medium Bioavailability	High Bioavailability
monotonous; very limited variety of foods	simple; limited variety of foods	wide variety of foods
high intake of cereals, roots, tubers etc.	high intake of cereals, roots, tubers etc.	high intake of meat, fish and/or vitamin C rich foods
minimal intake of meat, fish and/or vitamin C rich foods	some intake of meat, fish and/or vitamin C rich foods	

Bioavailability is greatly influenced by substances in the diet that may either enhance or inhibit absorption and utilization of dietary iron, particularly non-heme iron. For example, phytates found in whole grains (especially maize, millet, rice, wheat and sorghum), polyphenols (e.g., tannins found in legumes, tea, coffee), oxalates (found in green leafy vegetables) and calcium salts (found in milk products and tortillas prepared with calcium oxide) all inhibit iron absorption. Animal products (meat, poultry, fish and other seafood), vitamin C, and some food processing methods (fermentation and germination) all enhance the absorption of non-heme iron.

In developing countries, daily diets are low in animal products. They are typically based around a staple food high in unrefined carbohydrates, with legumes and vegetables accompanying the staple. This combination provides a diet of low iron bioavailability that is also high in inhibitors and low in enhancers of iron uptake. For example, analysis of the iron intake of pregnant women in rural Malawi showed that 89% of dietary iron was non-heme, and that the intake of bioavailable iron was significantly associated with iron status.[16] Similarly in rural Tanzania, assessment of typical household eating patterns revealed a largely grain and vegetable based diet, which although relatively high in total iron content, was very low in absorbable iron due to the presence of high levels of phytates and polyphenols.[17] An analysis of the diets of rural Bangladeshi women also found a very low heme iron intake coupled with high phytate intake, leading to a diet of poor iron bioavailability. Hemoglobin status was predicted by bioavailable iron in the diet, women's height and mid-upper-arm circumference and consumption of iron tablets, and more than half of the study subjects were anemic.[18]

Standard diets in industrialized countries are usually adequate to meet routine iron requirements of women, but are insufficient to supply the additional iron requirements of pregnancy. Thus in both developing and industrialized nations, iron supplementation, along with an optimum diet, is needed to prevent iron deficiency and anemia during pregnancy.

It is important to note that anemia is the final stage of iron deficiency, and that the preliminary phases, prior to a detectable drop in hemoglobin concentration, also have functional consequences such as reduced work productivity. Many individuals suffer from iron deficiency without reaching the severe iron depletion that causes anemia. In populations where iron deficiency anemia prevalence is of severe public health significance in a particular age and sex target group, all members of that group should be considered iron deficient and at risk of anemia.[19]

1.3.1.1. Interventions to Increase Iron Intake

The main interventions currently promoted and implemented to improve dietary iron intake include supplementation, fortification and dietary diversification and modification. Each of these has its strengths and limitations, which are discussed below.

Supplementation involves the provision of iron in tablet form to individuals or groups with or at risk for iron deficiency and anemia. The recommended dosing schedules for women are presented in Table 7.

**Table 7. Dosage Schedules for Iron Supplementation
to Prevent Iron Deficiency Anemia [20].**

Age Groups	Indications for supplementation	Dosage Schedule	Duration
Women of Childbearing Age	Where anemia prevalence is above 40%	Iron: 60 mg/day Folic acid: 400 μg/day	3 months
Pregnant Women	Universal supplementation	Iron: 60 mg/day Folic acid: 400 μg/day	As soon as possible after gestation starts – no later than 3rd month – and continuing for the rest of pregnancy
Lactating Women	Where anemia prevalence is above 40%	Iron: 60 mg/day Folic acid: 400 g/day	3 months post-partum

The most commonly implemented anemia control intervention is daily iron supplementation for pregnant women. This strategy is widely promoted as a key component of maternal health care in most countries. There is no doubt as to the *efficacy* of daily iron supplementation to improve maternal hemoglobin status in pregnancy, as demonstrated in many controlled trials.[21] However, the *effectiveness* of large-scale iron supplementation programs is questionable. For example, consistently high levels of maternal anemia were found in India (>80%) and Indonesia (>60%) through surveys conducted both before and after the introduction of iron supplementation programs[22]. A variety of constraints to effective large-scale supplementation programs for pregnant women have been identified, including irregular supply of tablets, limited access by women to health care services to obtain tablets, inadequate health counseling regarding the purpose and dosing regime of the supplements, and reluctance of women to consume the supplements.[23] These constraints can be overcome but a much higher level of supervision, training and support is required than is currently the norm in most places.

In addition, the importance of a lifecycle approach to anemia prevention and control is increasingly being recognized. Iron supplementation to pregnant women as a single anemia management strategy is likely to be ineffective, even if high coverage can be achieved, where pre-existing anemia prevalence (i.e., in non-pregnant women) is very high. This highlights the need to consider all women of childbearing age as a key target group for anemia prevention and control activities in high prevalence contexts. Iron supplementation will always be needed in pregnancy (as it is in industrialized nations), but if women enter pregnancy with adequate iron status the supplements consumed during pregnancy will be better able to maintain normal hemoglobin during a period of high demand for iron.[24]

While supplementation provides the best option for rapidly increasing hemoglobin concentration, it is not ideal as a long-term means of ensuring adequate iron status. Improving the dietary intake of bio-available iron through food-based approaches is key to sustainable prevention of iron deficiency anemia in developing countries. Food-based approaches include fortification, diversification of the diet, and modification of food preparation and consumption habits.

Fortification is the process of adding vitamins and/or minerals to a staple food in order to improve its nutritional value. There are many benefits to this approach, including the potential to fortify a single food with multiple micronutrients, thus addressing various dietary deficiencies with one intervention. In addition, fortification provides the opportunity to reach an entire population with improved nutrition, without requiring any change in dietary habits.

Development of a successful iron fortification program requires:

- identifying a suitable food vehicle which is consumed on a frequent basis by a significant proportion of the target population;
- technology for adding the iron to the food;
- social marketing to promote consumption of the food and explain the purpose of fortification;
- a quality control protocol to ensure that the food is fortified to consistent and safe levels.[25]

In many countries, national level initiatives provide increased dietary iron intake through fortification of staple foods and condiments by commercial or centralized processors. This approach is ideal in settings where the majority of the population purchases commercially processed food, and is highly cost-effective and sustainable.[26] However, in many developing countries a significant proportion of the population relies on subsistence farming and thus does not benefit from commercially fortified products. Efforts are being made to develop simple technologies to fortify foods at the community or household level in these contexts. One example of this type of fortification can be found in the description of anemia prevention activities implemented in Malawi, in the case study section of this chapter.

Dietary Diversification refers to interventions that promote an increase in the range and nutritional quality of foods consumed on a regular basis. One of the main contributors to nutritional deficiencies is consumption of a limited variety of foods. In the case of iron deficiency, low intake of animal source foods (which provide highly bioavailable heme iron) is of particular importance. In some contexts where vegetarianism is an important cultural or religious value, promoting animal source foods is not appropriate, but in most developing countries intake of animal foods is limited by poverty rather than beliefs. Much attention has been focused on supplementation and fortification as strategies to improve iron intake, but efforts to increase poor households' access to animal source foods are expanding. The case study section of this chapter provides an example of one such initiative, implemented in rural areas of Malawi. A major advantage of expanding dietary variety and quality through increased consumption of animal source foods is that an overall improvement in nutritional status and intake of essential vitamins and minerals is achieved.

In order to be effective in improving iron intake in vulnerable groups, dietary diversification activities must be geared towards household consumption of the animals raised rather than income generation through livestock sales. In addition, the selected animals must reproduce frequently enough to provide a regular source of meat, and must be culturally acceptable and able to thrive in the local environment. Inequitable distribution of food within households is a common risk to the success of dietary diversification programs, as in many cultures meat is preferentially served to men, with women consuming very little. However with delivery of carefully planned nutrition education messages, this constraint can be overcome.

Although animal source foods are of primary importance in efforts to improve dietary iron intake, dietary diversification interventions may also target increased vitamin C intake. Vitamin C is a potent enhancer of iron uptake by the body and is readily found in many fruits and vegetables. Supporting families to cultivate fruit trees and backyard gardens, combined with nutrition education on the importance of consuming vitamin C rich foods with meals, is another means of contributing to anemia reduction.

Dietary Modification is a term used to describe nutrition education initiatives aimed at changing the ways that foods are typically prepared, preserved and consumed, in order to improve the nutritional benefit of the diet. Small changes in traditional eating patterns can enhance uptake of available iron by the body. For example, tannins in tea and coffee can inhibit iron absorption, so these drinks should be consumed between rather than with meals in order to limit this effect. Germination and fermentation of grains can significantly increase iron bioavailability due to the breakdown of phytates, which are potent inhibitors of iron absorption. Limiting the cooking time of both iron-rich foods and vitamin C sources (fruits and vegetables) is also beneficial for improving iron uptake. These and other similar education messages related to maximizing iron bioavailability of the diet are an important component of improving iron status and reducing anemia prevalence.[27]

1.3.2. Other Nutritional Deficiencies

The presence of anemia often indicates broad spectrum nutritional inadequacy, not limited to insufficient iron intake alone. In particular, deficiencies of folic acid, vitamin A and vitamin B12 contribute to the development of anemia through their impact on red blood cell production. Since iron deficiency remains the dominant cause of anemia, promoting an overall improvement of dietary quality is an important approach to anemia prevention and control. For example, in a sample of 150 anemic pregnant women in Malawi, 55% were iron deficient but more than half of these had at least one other micronutrient deficiency as well. A further 26% had adequate iron status but were deficient in at least one other micronutrient, usually vitamin A.[28]

1.3.2.1. Interventions to Improve Micronutrient Status

The food-based interventions described above in relation to improving iron intake are also effective means of addressing other micronutrient deficiencies. For example, multiple micronutrients can be added as fortificants to staple foods. Increasing consumption of animal source foods increases intake of vitamin A, folic acid, vitamin B12 and many other essential nutrients in addition to iron. Supplementation is also used to meet women's needs for vitamin A, through the provision of high-dose capsules in the early post partum period, and folic acid is a standard component of iron supplements.

1.3.3. Malaria

Malarial infection leads to anemia through the destruction of red blood cells by the malaria parasites. Folate (folic acid) deficiency secondary to malaria can also develop as another cause of anemia. Malaria is a major cause of anemia in endemic areas, particularly in seasons of high transmission. One estimate suggests that 400,000 pregnant women in sub-Saharan Africa may develop severe anemia as a consequence of malaria infection in one year.[29] Malarial infection in pregnancy (although often asymptomatic) is a risk factor for maternal anemia as well as for delivery of a low birth weight infant and for anemia in the infant.[30]' [31] Primigravida women are most vulnerable, due to an apparent suppression of acquired immunity during the first pregnancy.[32] However, HIV infection is associated with greater malaria parasitemia among pregnant women of all parities.[33]

1.3.3.1. Interventions to Treat and Prevent Malaria in Pregnant Women

Intermittent Preventive Therapy refers to the provision of two doses of an anti-malarial drug (sulphadoxine-pyrimethamine) to women during pregnancy, through antenatal care services. Treatment of malaria in pregnancy by this method has been shown to reduce the prevalence of both severe maternal anemia[34] and low birth weight infants.[35] However, although intermittent preventive therapy is part of the national health policy of many countries, coverage is often low as many women have limited access to antenatal care services or do not seek care until late in pregnancy.

Insecticide-Treated Bed Net use is the key intervention for prevention of malaria infection and has demonstrated a positive effect on the prevalence of malaria and anemia in pregnant women.[36]. Distribution of nets to vulnerable groups is a major focus of the global strategy of the Roll Back Malaria Partnership.[37] As a result, provision of insecticide-treated nets to pregnant women is incorporated into routine antenatal services in many endemic countries.

Environmental Management to reduce the breeding grounds for mosquito larvae as well as larvicides can be part of a malaria prevention program where breeding sites are well defined.

1.3.4. Helminth Infections

Several species of worms contribute to anemia in developing countries, with hookworms and schistosomes being the most common. Both cause significant blood loss in the host, which leads to iron deficiency and anemia. An estimated one billion people worldwide are infected with hookworms, and although parasite control programs tend to focus on school children, women are also significantly affected and should be included in intervention programs[38]. For example, hookworm infection was identified as the strongest predictor of iron status in pregnant women in a study in rural Nepal, and anemia prevalence increased as intensity of hookworm infection increased[39].

1.3.4.1. Interventions to Control Helminth Infections

Antihelminthic Treatment, commonly known as deworming, is typically administered to school children in endemic areas. However it is also recommended that pregnant women in areas of high hookworm infection prevalence receive one dose of an antihelminthic medication after the first trimester.[40]

Improved Hygiene and Sanitation is an important component of helminth control. Use of latrines, hand washing, avoiding stagnant water and wearing shoes when walking outdoors all contribute to reduced risk of parasitic infection.

1.3.5. Chronic Infections

The relationship between infection and anemia varies with the nature of the disease. Chronic diarrheal disease and bacterial or viral infections of the gastrointestinal tract cause iron deficiency and anemia secondary to malabsorption and intestinal blood loss. Chronic inflammation is also associated with anemia due to swelling of tissues, rather than nutritional iron deficiency. Some diseases, such as tuberculosis, greatly increase metabolism, thus increasing the body's requirement for iron, and other nutrients and for overall caloric intake. These higher needs are often difficult to meet which leads to malnutrition, including the nutritional deficiencies which cause anemia.[41]

HIV infection is strongly linked with anemia through a variety of mechanisms. These include chronic disease and inflammation; increased metabolic and nutritional needs; poor intake of iron and other nutrients due to reduced appetite and anorexia; malabsorption of nutrients; and direct suppression of red blood cell production. Anemia is associated with disease progression and increased risk of death in HIV infected individuals.[42] In settings where anemia prevalence is already high due to chronic malnutrition, micronutrient deficiencies and helminth or malarial infections, HIV infection is likely to exacerbate pre-existing anemia through the additional effects of chronic inflammation and compromised immunity. For example, researchers in Malawi found that HIV-infection was significantly more prevalent in anemic pregnant women (47%) compared with the overall antenatal population (30%), and was associated with greater severity of anemia.[43] A study of HIV-infected pregnant women in Tanzania found that iron deficiency and infectious diseases (including malaria) were the main contributing factors to the observed high prevalence of anemia (83%, including 7% severe anemia)[44].

Interventions to treat infectious diseases vary according to the condition, and such a discussion is beyond the scope of this chapter. However, in addition to disease-specific treatment, optimizing the nutritional status of individuals suffering from chronic diseases is vital to anemia prevention as well as to improved immune function and recovery.

1.3.6. Reproductive Causes

The increased iron needs resulting from blood loss during menstruation and the demands of pregnancy make women particularly vulnerable to anemia. This risk is increased through frequent, closely spaced pregnancies, which do not allow time for maternal stores of iron and other nutrients to be replenished between pregnancies. Blood losses during childbirth and the post partum period also contribute to anemia in women, as do intrauterine contraceptive devices.[45]

1.3.7. Genetic Conditions

Hemoglobinopathies arising from genetic conditions such as sickle cell and thalassemia contribute to the burden of anemia in some regions of the world. Individuals with sickle cell disease (1-2% of sub-Saharan African infants) born in areas where health services are poor develop severe anemia in infancy and are unlikely to survive childhood, while those with sickle cell trait (30% of Africans) have altered hemoglobin production but are not at greater risk of severe anemia.[46]

1.3.8. Underlying Causes

The direct causes of anemia described in the preceding paragraphs are compounded by a variety of indirect factors, primarily related to poverty. These include food insecurity, which prevents consumption of a nutritionally adequate diet; lack of knowledge of anemia and its causes and prevention; poor hygiene and sanitation; and lack of access to health services. Thus the global burden of anemia is shouldered primarily by developing countries where resources are limited. However, there are effective interventions that can be implemented in resource-poor settings, dramatically reducing the prevalence of anemia in women and its associated morbidity, mortality and functional losses. Establishing comprehensive anemia control programs in high prevalence contexts is an urgent global health priority.

1.3.9 Multi-Factorial Etiology of Anemia

Anemia in women of developing countries is typically caused by iron deficiency plus one or more health issues. The relative contribution of these factors varies by geographic region and must be determined before effective interventions can be implemented.

For example, a study of anemia in pregnant women, non-pregnant women, adolescent girls and boys in an urban area of Tanzania found that iron deficiency was the main underlying cause of anemia in all groups, but that malaria and other infections were particularly common in pregnant women.[47] Another study conducted in a rural area of Tanzania also identified iron deficiency as the strongest predictor of anemia in women, but also found a significant association between anemia and malaria, schistosomiasis and hookworm infections.[48] An analysis of the etiology of anemia in pregnant women in rural Nepal found that 72.6% of the study subjects were anemic, and iron deficiency accounted for 88% of this anemia. However the strongest predictor of iron status was intensity of hookworm infection, with 74% of women affected. Infection with hookworm and *P. vivax* malaria were the strongest predictors of moderate to severe anemia, while low serum retinol (indicating vitamin A deficiency) was most strongly associated with mild anemia.[49] These studies illustrate the fact that although iron deficiency may be the primary cause of anemia, the disease factors contributing to depleted iron stores may vary and need to be assessed and addressed along with improving dietary iron intake.

1.4. Consequences of Anemia

Anemia in women leads to a variety of serious consequences, which are described below. These range from decreased work productivity and resulting economic losses, to maternal mortality. Anemia in pregnancy is also linked to adverse birth outcomes, thus contributing to an inter-generational cycle of poor health and compromised development.

1.4.1. Reduced Work Productivity

Hemoglobin transports oxygen in the blood for delivery to the body's tissues. Therefore one of the first signs of low hemoglobin, or anemia, is fatigue, due to lack of oxygen for physical activity. For the world's many anemic women, this causes work productivity and incomes to suffer, as well as the ability to carry out daily tasks and to nurture and care for children. The relationship between anemia and reduced productivity has been well documented. A literature review examining the association between iron deficiency and work capacity identified a strong causal effect of severe and moderate iron deficiency anemia on aerobic capacity, which translates into reduced physical activity and productivity.[50] Studies in a variety of countries have shown an improvement in work capacity for labourers in various occupations with the provision of iron supplementation.[51] A review of studies comparing work output in relation to changes in hemoglobin found consistent results across countries and contexts. A 10 percent increase in hemoglobin levels was associated with a 10 to 20 percent increase in work output.[52]

Given the clear relationship between iron deficiency anemia and reduced work capacity, there is value in improving iron status as a means of enhancing human capital, as well as for the health benefits to the individual. Anemia exacts a tremendous economic toll on developing countries. Anemia in young children is a widespread public health problem and is associated with irreversible cognitive deficits,[53] resulting in reduced wage-earning potential in adulthood. This effect, combined with labour losses from anemic adults in the workforce leads to significant economic losses. These have been estimated for several countries. The median cost has been estimated at $4 US per capita or approximately 0.9% of a developing country's GDP. South Asia bears the greatest actual loss – estimated at more than $5 billion annually - as the prevalence of anemia is highest and reliance on manual labour significant in this region.[54]

1.4.2. Increased Maternal Mortality

Severe anemia (Hb<7 g/dL) in pregnancy is associated with increased risk of maternal mortality. It has been estimated that the increased risk of death for pregnant women with Hb <7 g/dL is 1.35, and that those with Hb <5g/dL have a 3.5 times greater risk of dying from obstetric complications compared with non-anemic women.[55] A causal link between moderate anemia and maternal mortality has not yet been established, although the management of mild and moderate anemia is an important component of preventing the onset of severe anemia, which is directly linked to maternal deaths. However, broad-based interventions aimed at preventing or treating milder forms of anemia (such as iron supplementation) are unlikely to effectively address severe anemia. Saving mothers' lives through management of severe anemia requires a more focused and aggressive treatment approach.[56]

Estimates of the contribution of anemia to global maternal mortality vary, with suggested figures ranging from 67,500 [57] to 111,000 [58] maternal deaths per year. The World Bank estimates that approximately 10% of maternal deaths could be averted if full coverage of treatment for both iron deficiency anemia and malaria were to be implemented globally.[59]

1.4.3. Adverse Birth Outcomes

The results of several studies have shown an association between maternal iron deficiency anemia in early pregnancy and a greater risk of preterm delivery and consequent low birth weight. [60] Low birth weight greatly increases the risk of neonatal mortality and morbidity,[61] and is also associated with a variety of deficits in health, development and cognitive growth for the surviving infant. In addition, infants of anemic mothers have reduced iron stores continuing into the first year of life, increasing their vulnerability to iron deficiency and anemia.[62] This in turn contributes to compromised cognitive development in early childhood, even if the iron deficiency is corrected.

However, studies also show that abnormally high hemoglobin concentrations increase the risk of low birth weight and other adverse birth outcomes. This is caused by poor plasma volume expansion and hypertensive disorders of pregnancy, rather than iron status. Provision of supplementary iron in pregnancy will not elevate hemoglobin concentration above levels needed for optimum oxygen transport.[63]

1.5. Conclusion

Anemia is a widespread global public health problem. Women are particularly vulnerable, and more than half of all pregnant women in developing countries suffer from anemia. Iron deficiency is the primary cause, but a variety of other nutritional deficiencies and infectious diseases contribute significantly to the global burden of anemia. The consequences of anemia are serious and include economic losses, maternal mortality and adverse birth outcomes. A variety of interventions for anemia prevention and control are available, addressing all the major causes, but experience with effective program implementation has been limited. This issue is further explored in the remainder of the chapter.

2.0. PROGRAMS FOR ANEMIA PREVENTION AND CONTROL

2.1. Principles of Effective Programming

Despite the high prevalence of anemia and its serious consequences, very few examples of effective anemia control programs exist. This may be due to the multi-factorial etiology of anemia and the fact that there is not one easily administered solution available. Many individual interventions have been shown to be efficacious in research trials but when implemented on a wider scale in a non-controlled setting, they have typically not proven to be effective. This is particularly the case with iron supplementation, where issues of access, supply, compliance and poor health counseling regarding the purpose of the supplement have led to little change in anemia rates despite widespread implementation[64][65]

The lack of evidence of effective programs can lead to pessimism as to whether anemia really can be reduced on a wide scale. However the issue is not that appropriate interventions do not exist, but that the barriers to implementing them in an integrated manner in independent populations (as opposed to research settings) need to be better understood and overcome. The international community has made a renewed commitment to reducing anemia by one-third by 2010, and if this is to be achieved, it will require multiple interventions that target the various causes of anemia and also reach people at all levels of society. For example, commercial fortification of staple grains, condiments and other widely consumed products is an excellent strategy to increase iron intake of urban dwellers and other populations that purchase their food from commercial sources. However in settings where most people are subsistence farmers, this intervention will not have the desired impact, and other means of increasing iron intake, such as home-based fortification and raising of small animals, are needed.

In summary, the development of effective anemia control programming first requires analysis of the main determinants of anemia in the target population and then selection of interventions that are most likely to be effective given the socio-demographic characteristics of the intended beneficiaries. This is best accomplished through collaboration with multiple partners and integration of anemia control interventions with appropriate existing structures and services.[66],[67]

2.2. Program Examples

Although they are few in number, examples of this type of programming do exist. As early as the 1970s the government of Thailand identified anemia control as a national priority. Pregnant women were selected as the primary target group, and an improved system of antenatal care, including iron supplement distribution, was instituted using a network of village health volunteers. Logistical improvements ensured a regular supply of supplements and qualitative research was used to strengthen health counseling services regarding anemia and iron supplements. Although a comprehensive evaluation of the program has not been undertaken, National Nutrition Survey data indicates an impressive reduction in the prevalence of maternal anemia, from approximately 32-48% in the 1980s (depending on geographic region) to 8-28% by the late 1990s. [68] Thailand's anemia control strategy is now focusing on other target groups and additional interventions, such as weekly iron supplementation to school children and women of childbearing age (implemented through workplaces), and food fortification.

In Egypt, anemia prevalence among adolescents was reduced by 20% (from 30% to 24%) through a school-based program that provided weekly iron supplements and nutrition education to both girls and boys. These interventions were selected after it was determined that neither hookworm nor malaria was a major contributor to anemia in the target population. Control of schistosomiasis in school-aged children was already an existing intervention and so the anemia control program focused exclusively on iron deficiency, with significant success.[69]

In the 1990s the Malawi Maternal Anemia Control Program assessed the contributors to anemia among pregnant women in Thyolo District. The analysis showed that both socio-economic status (suggesting dietary factors) and malaria were linked to anemia, and so the project interventions focused on iron supplementation and improving antenatal care services (which included malaria prophylaxis). Follow-up evaluation showed that the prevalence of anemia had been significantly reduced in post partum women (those who delivered in the 6 months prior to the survey), from 61% to 51%. Anemia prevalence also decreased in pregnant women, but the change was not statistically significant. However women's intake of iron supplements greatly increased and antenatal care services improved as a result of the program, and the need for anemia control measures reached the national health agenda, paving the way for future initiatives.[70]

New endeavours that hold promise for reaching the international target of a 30% reduction in anemia by 2010 include the comprehensive approach currently being rolled out in five Central Asia countries. Kazakhstan, Uzbekistan, the Kyrgyz Republic, Turkmenistan and Tajikistan all share a common anemia prevention and control strategy that was developed in consultation with multiple partners. In line with the recommendation to address anemia through integration of key interventions, the strategy includes wheat flour fortification, iron supplementation to vulnerable groups, dietary diversification and nutrition education, and control of diseases such as malaria and helminth infections.[71] Although no evaluation results are available yet, this is a promising example of a multi-faceted, comprehensive approach to anemia control.

2.3. Conclusion

The current prevalence of anemia in women in developing countries is unacceptably high and a more intensive effort is required to address it. Although there are many challenges to the management of anemia, a few examples and models of successful initiatives do exist. Effective anemia prevention and control requires analysis of the main causes of anemia in the target population followed by implementation of a package of relevant interventions, integrated within existing structures and services, including health care, agriculture and education, and the private sector (e.g., food processing).

The final section of this chapter presents a more detailed case study of an anemia control program implemented in Malawi and Ghana, which demonstrates the principles of effective programming outlined above. As the other examples cited indicate, these principles can be applied in a wide range of program contexts, with positive results.

3.0. CASE STUDY: ANEMIA PREVENTION AND CONTROL IN GHANA AND MALAWI

3.1. Overview of MICAH Program

The MICronutrients And Health (MICAH) program was launched in 1995 by World Vision Canada with funding from the Canadian International Development Agency (CIDA). The goal of the program was to reduce the prevalence of micronutrient deficiencies in women and children, in line with international targets set at the 1990 World Summit for Children for the virtual elimination of vitamin A and iodine, and the reduction of iron deficiency anemia in women and children by one-third.

MICAH was implemented in five African countries (Ethiopia, Ghana, Malawi, Senegal and Tanzania) from 1996-2005. The first phase of the program (1996-2000) reached 3.8 million people, and the second phase (2001-2005) served a total beneficiary population of 2.7 million. The program design was based on the following characteristics:

- *Evidence based.* A baseline survey was conducted in each country to determine the major micronutrient deficiencies, target groups and priority intervention strategies. This led to context-specific program plans designed to address real needs. The program was monitored on a regular basis and was rigorously evaluated through cross-sectional surveys in 2000 and 2004.

- *Comprehensive.* MICAH partners implemented multiple interventions to address anemia and other micronutrient deficiencies. In addition, the program influenced micronutrient deficiency control at various levels, from advocacy for national policy change, to supporting village health volunteers to distribute iron supplements to empowering women in households to raise small animals.
- *Collaborative.* Although World Vision was the key implementing agency in each country, partnerships with government ministries and other agencies working in the fields of nutrition, health and agriculture were essential to the success of the program, and MICAH interventions were integrated into existing systems, structures and services. In Ethiopia and Malawi, partner organizations directly implemented the interventions in many locations.

Results from Ghana and Malawi are presented as examples of how these programming principles were applied in different contexts in order to reduce the prevalence of anemia in women.

4.0. GHANA

4.1. Background

The MICAH Program was implemented in 110 rural farming communities in the Kwahu West and Kwahu South Districts of the Eastern Region of Ghana, covering a total population of about 150,000. The District Health Management Team (DHMT) of the Ministry of Health selected the communities with consideration being given to those that were under-serviced and inaccessible to health staff, and where a high prevalence of anemia and goiter (evidence of iodine deficiency) had been identified. HIV prevalence is low in Ghana, with an estimated infection rate among adults of 3.1%,[72] so this was not a major influence on the effectiveness of MICAH interventions.

The MICAH activities were implemented in close collaboration with the Ghana Health Service, Ministry of Food and Agriculture, Ghana Education Service, Environmental Health Unit, Ministry of Local Government and the District Assemblies.

4.2. Anemia Prevention and Control Strategy

The key strategy implemented by MICAH Ghana for anemia control was iron/folic acid (IFA) supplementation to vulnerable groups. Dietary diversification activities were also implemented, including promotion of household gardens and raising small animals for meat consumption. Household gardening activities included the promotion of citrus fruits as a source of vitamin C to enhance iron absorption. However the raising of small animals, which has the potential to significantly increase dietary iron intake and absorption, was introduced later in the program lifetime, with limited coverage. Although some malaria prevention activities were undertaken (particularly environmental measures to reduce mosquito breeding grounds), the prevalence of malaria in women was found to be low during the baseline survey[73] (6.0% in non-pregnant women) and so was considered unlikely to be a major contributor to the high prevalence of anemia in women. Hookworm prevalence in school-aged children (a measure of infection burden in the overall population) was also low (4.4%) and so the anemia strategy focused primarily on improving iron intake through supplementation, with a minor emphasis on preventing malaria and hookworm.

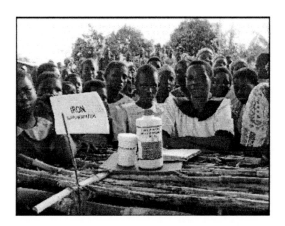

Two target groups were selected for iron supplementation: pregnant women, who received daily supplements through antenatal clinics, and non-pregnant women of childbearing age, who received weekly supplements through community health volunteers. Both these groups were included as a result of the baseline finding that anemia prevalence was at the level of a severe public health problem in all women, not just pregnant women.

The program achieved excellent coverage for IFA supplementation in both target groups and monitoring activities showed very high compliance rates. In fact, as women in the communities realized the benefits of improved hemoglobin levels, older women and men who were outside the target group for supplementation began to request IFA for themselves as well. This is a qualitative example of compliance and increased demand (beyond what the program could supply) for IFA supplements.

4.3. Methods of Evaluation of Program Effectiveness

The effectiveness of the MICAH program was evaluated through a series of cross-sectional surveys conducted at baseline in 1997, at mid-term in 2000 and at the close of the program in 2004. Multiple-indicator cluster survey methodology was followed. The 2000 and 2004 surveys included comparison groups from non-MICAH communities. Although these were not strict control groups they provide a basis of comparison with the neighbouring program areas. Further detail on the evaluation methodology is available in the final survey report.[74]

4.4. Results

The program was effective in decreasing the prevalence of anemia among pregnant and non-pregnant women, when compared both to initial levels and non-MICAH comparison areas (table 8). Indeed, over the seven years of the MICAH program, there was a 65% or two-thirds reduction of 1997 levels of anemia.

Table 8. MICAH Ghana Anemia Results in Women of Child Bearing Age and Pregnant Women, Comparing Baseline and Follow-up Surveys.

Indicator	Baseline Survey (1997)	Follow-up Survey (2000)		Final Survey (2004)	
	MICAH (n)	MICAH (n)	Non-MICAH (n)	MICAH (n)	Non-MICAH (n)
Women of child bearing age:					
Anemia prevalence (Hb<12g/dL)	47.9 (261)	26.9[*] (450)	38.0 (50)	16.1[*] (323)	32.3[**] (127)
Mean Hb ± SD (g/dL)	11.7 ± 1.8 (261)	12.8[*] ± 1.6 (450)	12.5 ± 1.5[*] (50)	12.9[*] ± 1.2 (323)	12.6 ± 1.4[**] (127)
IFA supplement coverage (weekly) (%)	NA	93.9 (380)	0[**] (43)	75.7 (309)	1.6[**] (124)
Attended Antenatal Clinic (during previous pregnancy) (%)	91.8 (282)	94.3 (420)	93.8 (48)	98.4 (309)	95.2[**] (124)
Malaria prevalence (%)	6.6 (259)	6.0 (385)	10.0 (50)	3.0[*] (304)	8.8[**] (125)
Have mosquito net (%)	NA	NA	NA	38.2 (309)	14.5[**] (124)
Pregnant women:					
Anemia prevalence (Hb<11g/dL)	60.0 (25)	48.4[*] (159)	NA	18.2[*] (383)	35.9[**] (159)
Mean Hb± SD (g/dL)	10.3 ± 2.6 (25)	11.0[*] ± 1.5 (159)	NA	12.1[*] ± 1.5 (383)	11.6 ± 1.7[**] (159)
IFA supplement coverage during current pregnancy (%)	21.7 (23)	69.7[*] (155)	NA	69.2[*] (380)	65.2 (155)
Attended Antenatal Clinic (during previous pregnancy) (%)	75.0 (24)	92.9 (156)	NA	96.3 (380)	90.3[**] (155)
Malaria prevalence (%)	4 (25)	6.6 (136)	NA	2.4 (363)	17.6[**] (153)
Have mosquito net (%)	NA	NA	NA	34.2 (380)	10.3[**] (155)
School Age children:					
Hookworm prevalence (%)	4.4 (182)	3.2[*] (354)	NA	0.8[*] (491)	0.8 (132)

[*] = p value <0.05 for test of statistical difference between baseline and follow-up

[**] = p-value <0.05 for test of statistical difference between MICAH and non-MICAH

This is twice the international target of reducing anemia by one-third. Anemia among women in the MICAH areas of Ghana moved from a severe public health range to a mild (non-pregnant) or moderate (pregnant) range. In the non-MICAH comparison areas, the prevalence of anemia remained at the high end of the moderate range in both pregnant and non-pregnant women.

In addition to the overall reduction in anemia prevalence in MICAH areas, figures 1 and 2 show the shift in relative proportion of mild, moderate and severe anemia over the program lifetime.

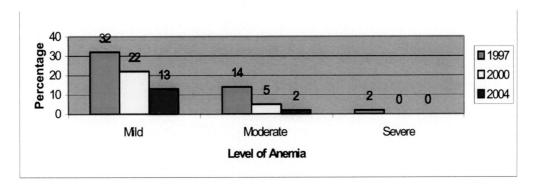

Figure 1. Anemia in women of child bearing age Ghana, MICAH.

The clear trend of decreasing anemia prevalence is also reflected in the distribution of hemoglobin values. As figures 3 and 4 illustrate, the distribution curves for both pregnant and non-pregnant women in MICAH areas shifted markedly to the right (higher Hb levels) over the course of the program.

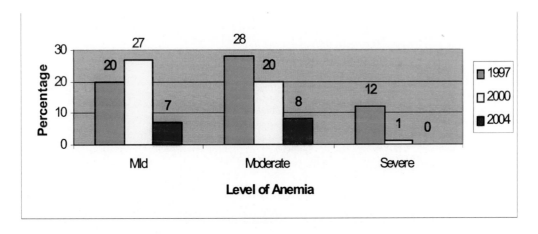

Figure 2. Annemia in pregnant women Ghana, MICAH.

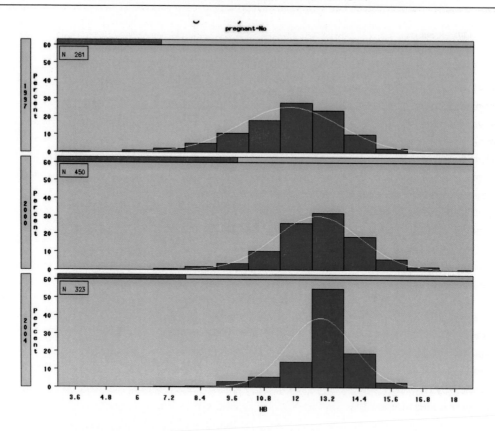

Figure 3. Distribution of hemoglobin by year within MICHA communities.

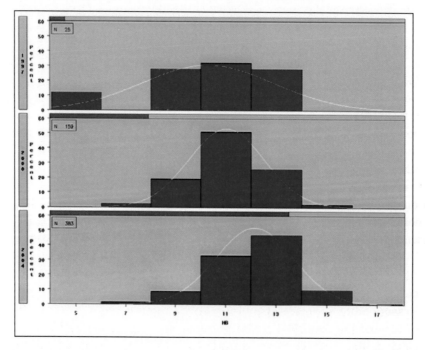

Figure 4. Distribution of hemoglobin by year within MICHA communities.

4.5. Discussion

Two key observations from the MICAH Ghana experience provide useful lessons that may inform anemia control efforts in other settings. The first is that weekly IFA supplementation can be effectively implemented, reducing the prevalence of anemia in non-pregnant women. The second is that although coverage of IFA supplements to pregnant women was very high in both MICAH and non-MICAH areas in 2004, anemia rates were significantly lower in the MICAH areas, where women had received regular iron supplementation prior to becoming pregnant. This suggests that where anemia is in the severe public health range among non-pregnant women, provision of IFA only during pregnancy is insufficient to prevent maternal anemia. These two issues are discussed below in further detail.

4.5.1. Weekly Iron Supplementation is an Effective Means of Reducing the Prevalence of Anemia in Non-Pregnant Women of Childbearing Age

Extensive debate has taken place in the scientific community regarding the relative efficacy and effectiveness of daily versus intermittent (i.e. weekly) iron supplementation to high-risk groups. A review of available evidence led to the conclusion that daily supplementation remains the intervention of choice for anemia control in pregnant women.[75] However, the potential for weekly iron supplementation as an anemia prevention and control measure in other vulnerable groups continues to be explored, with many positive results. It may be that ultimately the issue of feasibility of supervision to ensure compliance will be what determines the benefit of one supplementation regime over another[76]

Weekly IFA supplementation to women of childbearing age, along with increased prevention of malaria, through MICAH Ghana led to a 66% reduction in the prevalence of anemia in this group (from 48% to 16%) over the seven year program lifetime. By 2004 the prevalence of anemia was significantly lower in the MICAH (16%) compared with non-MICAH (32%) areas. The MICAH experience demonstrates that operational challenges to effective, long-term supplementation programs for anemia prevention can be overcome, with impressive results.

In order to accomplish this, MICAH Ghana implemented a well-planned approach to IFA distribution, designed to address the major points of weaknesses in many IFA supplementation initiatives. The typical limitations of such programs include irregular supply of tablets, inadequate supervision, and lack of appropriate health counseling regarding the supplements. However these common barriers were well managed in the MICAH approach and did not compromise results. The main contributors to the successful coverage of IFA supplementation to non-pregnant women in MICAH Ghana include the following:

- *Integration within existing health system.* The MICAH program relied on a strong partnership with the Ministry of Health at the district and sub-district levels. Responsibility for distribution of IFA supplements was integrated into the mandate of the existing Sub-District Health Teams, who provide a variety of maternal and child health services to the communities. However additional support for IFA supplementation was provided by a network of community health volunteers (CHVs) established by MICAH. The CHVs worked closely with the Sub-District

Health Teams and were supervised by the Ministry of Health staff. MICAH provided regular training and capacity building opportunities for the CHVs, particularly related to counseling women regarding the importance, purpose and correct dosing of the IFA tablets.

- *Community-based distribution.* Using the network of CHVs, the program was able to provide IFA supplements to women within their own communities. This is a key aspect of achieving high coverage with routine supplementation. Compliance rates tend to drop dramatically if women are not able to access the supplements in their home area but must travel to obtain them. In MICAH Ghana, women would come to local distribution points and collect a month's supply of IFA supplements at a time. The CHVs were given small incentives on an annual basis in recognition of their work, and their role was key to the success of the weekly IFA supplementation for women of childbearing age.

- *Management of supply and logistics.* The MICAH program was responsible for ordering IFA tablets on a semi-annual basis and ensuring their distribution to the sub-district level through the Ministry of Health system. Shortages in the supply of tablets was not an issue. However it is a concern for the future, as the sustainability of the intervention following the close of MICAH depends on reassignment of responsibility for managing the supply of tablets, as well as funding for their purchase. Advocacy for funding to ensure the continuation of routine IFA supplementation is being undertaken. Given the high economic costs of anemia to developing countries, the investment of core health care funding in a proven effective anemia prevention and control strategy would yield a high return.

- *Effective behaviour change communication.* The program included a strong nutrition education component, particularly at the community level. Messages regarding the causes and consequences of anemia and the importance of women taking regular IFA tablets were disseminated through a variety of culturally appropriate avenues. These included radio talks and presentations in mosques, churches, and marketplaces. The nutrition education activities included clear information aimed at improving compliance to IFA supplementation, such as descriptions of possible side effects and ways to manage them, and tips for remembering to take the tablets according to the dosing schedule.

Although contexts vary and creativity to adapt to local conditions is always needed in the development of effective health programs, inclusion of the factors outlined above is key to effective IFA supplementation programming. With careful planning and strong partnerships, the common failures of supplementation programs can be avoided, and the prevalence of anemia in non-pregnant women of childbearing age can be significantly reduced.

4.5.2. High IFA Coverage to Pregnant Women does not Effectively Reduce Maternal Anemia Prevalence When Pre-Existing Levels of Anemia are in the Severe Public Health Range

There was a significant decrease in anemia in pregnant women in MICAH areas, from 60% at baseline to 18% in 2004. At the same time, IFA coverage significantly increased from 22% to 69% in MICAH areas. In non-MICAH comparison areas IFA supplementation coverage was similarly high (65%) at the time of the final survey, but anemia prevalence was much greater (36%).

The difference in anemia prevalence rates may be partly due to the much higher prevalence of malaria among pregnant women in the non-MICAH areas (18%) compared with MICAH areas (2%).[77] The lower prevalence of malaria in the MICAH areas may have been due to higher mosquito net coverage (34% vs. 10% in non-MICAH areas). Coverage of anti-malarial medication (IPT) to pregnant women was significantly higher (p=0.04) in MICAH areas (61.5%) compared with non-MICAH (54.5%), but in both groups coverage of this intervention was greater than 50%.

However, notwithstanding the contribution of malaria, iron deficiency is likely to be the major cause of anemia in pregnant women in non-MICAH areas. This is typical in developing countries and was shown to be the case in the MICAH areas through the effective use of IFA supplementation to address anemia. The comparison between anemia rates and IFA coverage for pregnant women in MICAH and non-MICAH areas at the final survey strongly suggest that provision of IFA supplementation only to pregnant women is not an effective means of controlling maternal anemia in settings where anemia prevalence is in the range of a severe public health problem in all women of childbearing age. Given the body's additional demand for iron in pregnancy, it is unreasonable to expect that women entering pregnancy in an anemic or iron deficient state will be able to attain and maintain normal hemoglobin status even with high compliance to a daily IFA supplementation regime.

The international health community is increasingly adopting a lifecycle approach to anemia prevention and control. This includes the recognition that pre-existing iron deficiency or anemia is difficult to correct in pregnancy, and that reducing the widespread prevalence of maternal anemia requires improved iron intake in adolescent girls and women of childbearing age prior to first pregnancy, [78] in addition to the recommended universal daily IFA supplementation during pregnancy.[79] Weekly IFA supplementation to non-pregnant women followed by daily IFA supplementation during pregnancy, while also implementing measures to prevent malaria, can effectively reduce anemia in pregnancy, as the MICAH Ghana experience demonstrates. Similar results have been reported in other contexts. For example, a social marketing initiative in Vietnam promoted weekly IFA supplementation to women of childbearing age, with the result that when the women became pregnant, their hemoglobin levels were maintained at normal levels in the first two trimesters, and the prevalence of low birth weight infants was minimal.[80]

4.6. Conclusion

One of the chief limitations of IFA supplementation as a strategy for anemia prevention is the difficulty of effectively programming the intervention on a wide scale.[81] Issues of supervision, which include ensuring both regular supply of tablets and women's compliance with the supplementation regime, have frequently been cited as reasons for the ineffectiveness of many large-scale IFA supplementation initiatives.[82] However, where iron deficiency anemia is a severe public health problem, IFA supplementation still offers one of the most efficacious means of improving hemoglobin status in both pre-pregnant and pregnant women. Women of childbearing age are an important target group for supplementation in areas where anemia prevalence is in the severe public health range. Improving women's iron status prior to pregnancy, followed by daily iron supplementation to maintain normal hemoglobin status during pregnancy, can significantly reduce maternal anemia and its associated consequences.

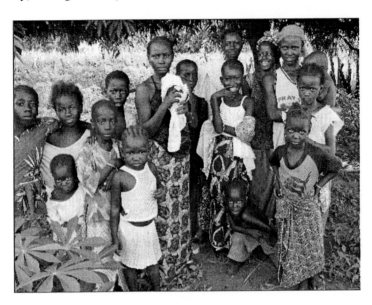

The experience of MICAH Ghana shows that the implementation challenges to providing routine IFA supplementation to women of childbearing age can be overcome if existing local systems and structures are appropriately utilized. In rural Ghana this involved strong partnership with the Ministry of Health and mobilization of a network of community health volunteers, but in other settings it may be more appropriate to deliver IFA through avenues such as workplaces or the private sector.[83] In Indonesia, the Ministry of Health and MotherCare project used marriage registries to reach young women with messages about IFA supplementation. Follow-up monitoring after 3-4 months of the intervention showed that anemia prevalence in the newly married women had decreased by 40%, from 23.8% at baseline to 14.0%.[84] More of this kind of innovative, context-specific approach to delivery systems for IFA supplementation to women of childbearing age is urgently needed as part of the global effort to reduce anemia.

5.0. MALAWI

5.1. Background

Malawi is one of the world's poorest countries, with a largely rural population reliant on subsistence farming for survival. Large regions of the country are affected by recurrent drought, and in recent years HIV prevalence has dramatically increased. Official estimates suggest over 14% of the adult population is infected with HIV,[85] and a higher level of seropositivity (30%) has been identified in pregnant women.[86] As in other southern African countries, the HIV/AIDS epidemic has left a devastating impact on the labour force and social structure in Malawi.

The MICAH program was implemented in all three regions of Malawi (north, central and south), targeting1.8 million people. The program operated in 19 project sites, covering 14 of the 26 districts in the country. The program operated largely in the rural areas, where people are mainly subsistent farmers, growing crops of maize and beans. The selected project areas reflected expressed needs by communities, with assistance from government line ministries and assessment by the World Vision field staff in the areas. Proposals were submitted to the World Vision Malawi MICAH office for consideration and were funded if they met the set criteria of the steering committee.

Key program partners included government institutions such as the Agriculture Development Divisions (ADDs) of the Ministry of Agriculture and Irrigation, the Ministry of Health and Population (MOHP), and the Community Health Sciences Unit (CHSU). Other partner agencies included non–governmental organizations (NGOs) operating in the health and agriculture sectors, and mission hospitals.

5.2. Anemia Prevention and Control Strategy

A cross-sectional baseline survey at the start of the MICAH program confirmed the presence of significant levels of anemia and malaria (59 and 24 percent, respectively) in pregnant women, and intestinal parasites (20% hookworm) in school aged children (see tables 9,10). Based on these findings, the program design included a comprehensive package of interventions to address the contributors to anemia. As the major contributor to anemia in Africa is known to be iron deficiency, a major component of the program thus included a variety of interventions to increase the intake and bioavailability of iron such as, iron supplements (weekly to all women of child-bearing age and daily to pregnant women); increasing iron-rich foods and iron enhancers (e.g., animal foods, citrus fruits); food processing methods (e.g., soaking maize to decrease phytate); and fortifying staple foods (i.e., maize) with iron. In addition, the program included interventions to decrease diseases affecting anemia (e.g., malaria prevention and treatment; construction and use of latrines), as well as capacity building and advocacy for improved anemia programs at all government levels.

These interventions were integrated into existing community structures and services, in partnership with relevant government agencies and other groups as follows.

Interventions to Increase Iron intake:

- *Iron supplements* were provided daily at the community level to pregnant women through Traditional Birth Attendants (TBAs), and weekly to all women of childbearing age through trained Community Health Volunteers (CHVs). In order to ensure high compliance rates, the iron tablets were consumed in front of the CHVs and TBAs, who maintained register books with detailed records of each woman's supplement intake.
- *Dietary diversification* was a key component of MICAH Malawi's anemia control strategy. The typical diet in rural Malawi is very low in animal products and based on maize as a staple grain, which is very high in phytate, a potent inhibitor of iron absorption. MICAH Malawi intervened to increase household availability of animal

foods for consumption by women through training and start-up assistance for small animal revolving schemes.

By the end of the program in 2005, over 63% of total MICAH population reared and consumed small animals and fowl. The initial distribution of 36,243 animals resulted in revolving an additional 15,213 animals by end of program.

A revolving scheme is a distribution method whereby the program provides initial animal stock to a number of individuals who have been selected according to criteria determined with the community. These individuals then give the first offspring from their animals to others in the community, and so on until full distribution is achieved. The beneficiaries were required to construct a shelter to house the animals or birds, according to training provided by staff from the Ministry of Agriculture Department of Veterinary Services. The animals included goats (initially), rabbits, chickens and guinea fowl. However, the accompanying nutrition education promoted the consumption of all animal source foods.

Initially the program focused on goats, by providing an improved variety of male goats for breeding with traditional local female goats to produce offspring with better meat and milk production potential. However a mid-term evaluation revealed that because goats are relatively large and important animals within the community setting, they were not being consumed on a regular basis by households, and were not under the control of the women, who provided meals for the household. Rather, they would be used for ceremonial purposes such as for a chief's wedding or funeral or major religious events. At these events, it was usually the men that would consume the meat and women would often only receive a small portion, if any at all. It was thus concluded that although the goats were valued as an input by the communities, the intervention was not directly contributing to an increase in women's consumption of animal source foods.

Through collaboration and discussion with the Ministries of Agriculture and Health and the MICAH implementing partners, the promotion of rabbits was identified as a possible means of improving the quality of dietary intake within the target area. Rabbits are small and therefore not as highly valued as the larger goats. Also, rabbits reproduce quickly, unlike the one goat kid per year, and were thus used by women for family meals. The lower perceived value of the rabbits also enabled the women to have decision-making control over the use of the rabbits, whereas the goats were under the control of the male household head.

Since the consumption of rabbit meat was new to most project communities, significant effort was required in introducing the concept. Cooking demonstrations and taste-tests involving influential members of the communities, particularly religious leaders, proved an effective means of overcoming initial hesitation regarding the rabbits. The staff also assessed each community to decide on the committee that would take up the responsibility of the rabbit revolving funds and identification of initial beneficiaries. In some cases, the initial beneficiary was the chief's household, or another influential member of the community. This was due to the fact that once these influential people adopted the new practice of rabbit rearing, it would be deemed acceptable by the others. In other cases, especially needy families would be identified as primary beneficiaries so that the community would be able to see the difference made in the diet and lives of the even people with few resources. In this way, the program adapted to the unique characteristics of each community in order to maximize the acceptance and coverage of the dietary diversification interventions.

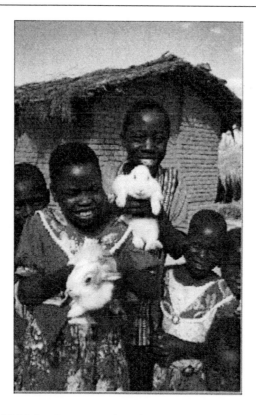

In addition, MICAH Malawi promoted and supported the establishment of gardens at most households (final survey showed 55% of households with a garden) and 64 communal gardens, in close collaboration with the Ministry of Agriculture and Irrigation. The emphasis was on cultivation of fruits that enhance iron absorption through vitamin C (such as citrus fruits) or that are rich in vitamin A (mango, papaya), and dark green leafy vegetables from indigenous varieties. Solar driers were introduced as a best practice in preservation of fruits and vegetables, to provide a year-round source of micronutrients.

Fortification was pilot-tested in MICAH Malawi through the addition of a micronutrient premix during grinding at the village mills. In rural Malawi, maize is grown on small plots by individual families and then brought by the women to village mills for grinding. Thus, the process of developing small scale fortification involved extensive consultation with local and international experts, experimentation with various methods of adding the micronutrient premix, and establishment of a strong partnership with the private sector (village mill owners and operators).

Effective communication to all stakeholders, particularly to the community members, was essential for acceptance of the fortified maize. During the initial start-up of the fortification services in any given project area, the community would be introduced to the concept of fortification through various media. Drama groups would make vivid demonstrations of the benefits of the fortified flour and how to fortify flour. Taste-testing competitions and cooking demonstrations enabled the community to try the fortified flour to demonstrate that there would be no changes in organoleptic properties. In communities where there was continued resistance to accept fortified flour, specific targeted messages were developed to address the key points of misconception. Also, project staff identified influential people in the community and targeted messages there.

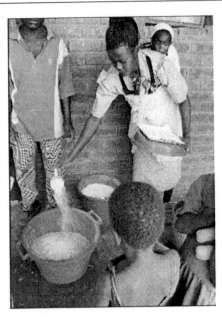

After initial positive results, the intervention was expanded to cover 19 community mills, servicing approximately 8,000 households. By the end of the MICAH program, over twice as many households in the MICAH areas (13.8%) were using fortified flour than in the comparison areas (6.3%). Furthermore, the experience of pioneering the small scale fortification process in Malawi resulted in the MICAH program earning a good reputation with the national government. This was partly reflected in the fact that, when the National Fortification Alliance was formed, World Vision was the only NGO invited to be a member. The small scale fortification project started by MICAH was included as part of the National Fortification Program, and the MICAH experience helped shape the direction of the Alliance in establishing a fortification strategy for Malawi.

Interventions to reduce prevalence of Diseases Affecting Anemia:

Malaria:

- MICAH supported *malaria prophylaxis* for pregnant women through distribution of anti-malarials to pregnant women, in collaboration with local health facilities. This was accomplished in large part by creating *Drug Revolving Fund* (DRF) schemes in project villages.
- Community committees were formed and trained to operate and manage these DRFs, which increased accessibility to *treatment for malaria* and other common illnesses, at the community level.
- MICAH provided training in prevention of malaria, which included establishment of revolving funds for *insecticide treated mosquito nets (ITNs)* and training in re-treating of mosquito nets. The ITN revolving funds were part of the DRFs, and ITNs were purchased by MICAH for the DRFs. The ITNs were resold to general community members, sold at subsidized prices to pregnant women and women with children under five, and provided free of charge to those who were the poorest in the communities.

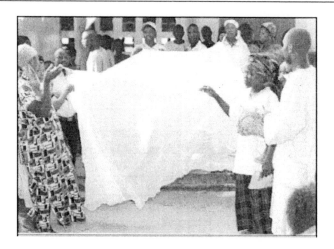

Prevention of Other Diseases (e.g., Helminth infections and schistosomiasis)

- *Environmental sanitation*: MICAH promoted the construction and use of latrines, garbage waste disposal and construction of utensil drying racks. Village Health Volunteers took the lead role to promote these activities in their own villages and communities. This strategy was very successful and resulted in the construction of over 12,000 pit latrines during the MICAH intervention period. In addition, communities were assisted to reduce schistosomiasis risk through clearing of bushes where snails tend to reproduce. The MICAH program also supported construction and maintenance of safe water supplies for households and schools.

Interventions to increase Capacity :

- Advocacy and Capacity Building. MICAH influenced the creation of the 'National Micronutrient Coordinator' position, housed in the Ministry of Health and Population and funded through the MICAH program. Advocacy through the Coordinator's office focused on national policy on anemia prevention, and national strategies for reducing anemia such as commercial scale fortification of maize flour. In addition, the National Micronutrient Coordinator and the MICAH Program Manager were members of the National Micronutrient Task Force. This group also influences policies in the country, such as the National Action Plan for Nutrition and the Poverty Reduction Strategy Paper, which included specific strategies and program guidelines for addressing anemia.

MICAH increased capacity at national, regional and community levels by including two line ministries (MOHP and MOAI) as implementing partners. This strong collaboration between MICAH and the government enhanced program influence by presenting a united approach to nutrition and health. MICAH also provided extensive capacity building to government staff and community workers and volunteers.

5.3. Methods of Evaluating the Program Effectiveness

As in Ghana, the effectiveness of the MICAH program in Malawi was evaluated through a series of cross-sectional surveys, conducted in 1997, 2000 and 2004. Multiple-indicator cluster survey methodology was followed. Details on evaluation methodology are available in the final survey report.[87]

In late 1999, an external mid-term evaluation recommended focusing more resources on fewer communities. As a result, MICAH Malawi scaled back the program implementation area. The areas chosen to continue with a more resource-intensive MICAH program were communities rated the poorest and most disadvantaged by the District Health Offices, and with the highest rates of malnutrition and communicable diseases. The remaining communities, where MICAH program interventions had been implemented for one year only, were then considered a 'Comparison' group in the 2000 and 2004 surveys. Those that continued to receive a full complement of MICAH interventions were considered 'MICAH' communities/clusters. Thus, by opportunistic criteria, an internal control group was identified. The inclusion of an internal control group allowed for a plausibility assessment of the program, and the different intensities of exposure to the program allows a stronger plausibility statement than findings from comparison between all and nothing groups.[88]

5.4. Results

The effectiveness of the MICAH program in improving hemoglobin (Hb) levels was evidenced among non-pregnant women by significant increased Hb levels in the MICAH communities from 2000 (11.8 ±1.7 g/dL) to 2004 (12.3±1.3 g/dL) while no change was observed in the Comparison areas (table 9).

Table 9. MICAH Malawi Anemia Results in Women of Child Bearing Age and Pregnant Women, Comparing Baseline and Follow-up and Final Surveys.

Indicator	Baseline Survey (1996)	Follow-up Survey (2000)		Final Survey (2004)	
		MICAH (n)	Comparison (n)	MICAH (n)	Comparison (n)
Women of child bearing age: Anemia prevalence (%) (Hb<12.0 g/dL)	NA	50.5 (1559)	45.7 (1442)	39.1 (1610)	44.9 (795)
Mean Hb ± SD (g/dL)	NA	11.8 ± 1.7 (1559)	12.0^ ± 1.7 (1442)	12.3** ± 1.3 (536)	12.1 ± 1.7^ (795)
Pregnant Women: Anemia prevalence (%) (Hb<11g/dL)	59.0 (417)	43.0* (156)	44.6* (175)	48.1 (208)	57.3 (89)
Mean Hb ± SD (g/dL)	10.3 ± 1.7 (417)	10.9* ± 1.5 (156)	11.0* ± 1.7 (175)	11.0* ± 1.5 (208)	10.8* ± 1.6 (89)

* = p value <0.05 for test of statistical difference between baseline and follow-up (2000) or final (2004)
** = p-value <0.05 for test of statistical difference between follow-up (2000) and final (2004)
^ = p-value <0.05 for test of statistical difference between MICAH and Comparison

Moreover, mean hemoglobin levels were significantly higher in MICAH than Comparison areas in 2004, while they were significantly lower than comparison areas in 2000. The significant interaction of MICAH and Comparison areas by year is illustrated in Graph 1.

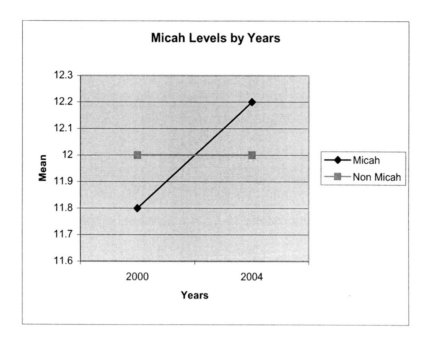

Figure 5. Mean Hemoglobin of Malawian women (non-pregnant) in the Micah and Comparison groups by year (2000 and 2004).

A trend corresponding to hemoglobin results was observed by decreased prevalence of anemia in MICAH Malawi program areas, from 2000 (50.5%) to 2004 (39.1%), compared with no change in the Comparison areas (table 9). Although not statistically significant, the reduction by 23% of 2000 levels of anemia, over a four-year period, is programmatically impressive, and approaches the international target of reducing anemia by one-third. Unfortunately, anemia was not evaluated at baseline for women of childbearing age.

In this same group, MICAH interventions, including coverage of weekly iron-folic acid (IFA) supplements and ITNs, increased between 2000 and 2004, and presence of small animals and fortified flour was significantly higher in MICAH than Comparison communities in 2004 (table 10).

Among pregnant women, there was a 27% decrease in anemia in MICAH areas from 1996 (59%) to 2000 (43.0%) but no further statistically significant change by 2004 (48.1%) (table 9). A corresponding improvement was observed in the hemoglobin levels, from 1996 to 2000, with no change occurring in 2004 (table 9). In contrast, although Comparison areas also underwent a significant decrease from 1997 (59%) to 2000 (45%), there was a close to significant (p=0.07) increase in anemia in 2004 (57.3%).

In pregnant women, MICAH interventions including coverage of daily IFA and ITNs increased within the MICAH communities from 1996 to 2000 and again to 2004, as well as being higher in the MICAH than Comparison communities in 2004 (table 10).

Hookworm prevalence decreased in school aged children over the program period in all groups. This was used as a proxy indicator for hookworm in women and indicated that hookworm was no longer a significant problem in these communities.

Table 10. Coverage of MICAH Malawi Interventions to address Anemia Women (non-pregnant and pregnant), Comparing Baseline and Follow-up and Final Surveys.

Indicator	Baseline Survey (1996)	Follow-up Survey (2000)		Final Survey (2004)	
		MICAH (n)	Comparison (n)	MICAH (n)	Comparison (n)
Women of child bearing age:					
INCREASING DIETARY IRON: Coverage of **weekly** IFA supplements (%)	NA	68.5 (1565)	13.2^ (1276)	93.5** (1294)	25.1**^ (747)
Presence of small animals (% of households)	42.8 (1269)	61.9* (1900)	48.8*^ (1802)	63.9* (1582)	50.6*^ (856)
Presence of fortified flour (% of households)	NA	NA	NA	13.8 (1582)	6.3^ (856)
CONTROL OF PARASITES: Malaria prevalence (%)	NA	21.8 (1603)	11.2^ (1477)	5.7** (1382)	5.1** (766)
Households with mosquito nets (%)	NA	11.1 (1575)	4.6^ (1337)	75.5** (1370)	58.1**^ (754)
Presence of latrine (% of households)	70.7 (1268)	89.3* (893)	82.1*^ (1697)	93.6* (1569)	93.3* (847)
Pregnant Women:					
INCREASING DIETARY IRON: Coverage of **daily** IFA supplements (% in current pregnancy)	40.0 (168)	69.6* (289)	34.7^ (300)	91.9*** (173)	74.4*^ (82)
CONTROL OF PARASITES: Malaria prevalence (%)	23.1 (385)	16.8* (297)	15.9* (327)	6.6*** (182)	6.0*** (84)
Households with mosquito nets (%)	3.6 (168)	13.4* (284)	2.4^ (289)	69.0*** (184)	51.9***^ (81)
School Aged Children:					
Hookworm prevalence (%)	20.2 (690)	10.6* (1094)	6.2* (1029)	0.0** (1019)	1.5** (506)

* = p value <0.05 for test of statistical difference between baseline and follow-up (2000) or final (2004)

** = p-value <0.05 for test of statistical difference between follow-up (2000) and final (2004)

^ = p-value <0.05 for test of statistical difference between MICAH and Comparison

In addition to comparing changes in prevalence of these indicators over time and between MICAH and Comparison groups, further statistical analysis of the MICAH Malawi data was performed to determine the association between various factors and mean hemoglobin levels in both pregnant and non-pregnant women. The full 2000 and 2004 data sets were combined for this analysis, thus findings presented in table 11 identify which factors associated with higher hemoglobin levels in Malawian women. Absence of malaria, presence of small animals, having a latrine, literacy, taking iron supplements (weekly), and clean drinking water are all factors positively affecting non-pregnant women's hemoglobin. Absence of malaria, taking iron supplements (daily), and having a latrine are factors positively associated with pregnant women's hemoglobin levels.

Table 11. Factors Associated with Higher Mean
Hemoglobin Levels in Malawian Women.

	Non-Pregnant Women	Pregnant Women
Not infected with malaria	√	√
Having small animals at the household	√	
Taking iron supplements	√	√
Having a household latrine	√	√
Able to read and write	√	
Clean drinking water in dry season	√	
Clean drinking water in rainy season	√	

5.5. Discussion

Two themes additional to those noted in the Ghana case study, emerge from MICAH Malawi's experience that may further inform anemia control efforts in similar settings. The first is that, despite the more challenging environment for anemia control in Malawi than in Ghana, progress can be made in reducing anemia. The second is that, the multiple factors associated with increased hemoglobin levels suggest that multiple interventions are essential to address anemia in the context of the multi-faceted etiology of anemia in Malawian women. These two issues are discussed below in further detail.

5.5.1. Anemia Prevalence Can Be Reduced Even in Settings with Significant Constraints Such as High HIV Prevalence and Drought

The improvements in hemoglobin and reductions in anemia seen in non-pregnant women in MICAH communities are not as substantial as the changes observed in MICAH Ghana. However the context in Malawi is considerably more challenging. In addition to chronic poverty, Malawians face recurrent drought and high HIV prevalence, both of which have the potential to compromise the effectiveness of anemia prevention and control activities.

During the intervention period, a major drought in Malawi took place in the 2001/2002 maize growing season. In order to cope with the severe food shortage, households were forced to sell valuable resources in order to find food. This included the small animals distributed as part of the MICAH program, which were either sold to get money to buy maize, or were consumed. In normal circumstances, at least a breeding pair would be kept, but in such a times of severe food shortage, hunger and malnutrition, all resources available were used in order to survive. There were many hunger-related deaths reported in Malawi during this season. Although the MICAH program did not collect nutrition data during the drought period, it is assumed that levels of malnutrition of all types, including anemia, either did not improve or deteriorated during this crisis, and that recovery and nutritional repletion afterwards would require a significant period of time, as well as inputs from external programs such as the MICAH program. This assumption is supported by the fact that in Comparison areas, between 2000 and 2004, the mean hemoglobin did not increase nor did the prevalence of anemia decrease among non-pregnant women (table 9), while anemia increased among pregnant women.

However, in the MICAH areas, the mean hemoglobin of non-pregnant women increased over this period and with a 22% decrease in anemia. The MICAH program launched an intensive animal restocking program in 2002-2003, and by the final program survey in 2004, 64% of households in the program area had small animals, similar to the level achieved prior to the drought (62%) (table 10). In addition, the MICAH program continued with the integrated multiple interventions, including distribution of weekly iron supplements, fortified maize flour, distribution of insecticide treated nets, and treatment and prevention of other parasites, all of which had higher coverage in MICAH areas than non-MICAH (table 10). It is possible that a greater reduction in anemia prevalence could have been achieved had the major setback of this food crisis not occurred.

As discussed in the first section of this chapter, HIV infection contributes both directly and indirectly to anemia. Anemia prevalence has been found to be much higher among HIV positive pregnant women in Malawi, compared with the overall antenatal population.[1] Thus the challenge of controlling maternal anemia in a high HIV prevalence context is intensified. The MICAH surveys did not assess HIV status of respondents, but considering the high HIV prevalence in the country and particularly among pregnant women, it is more than reasonable to consider it a major confounding factor, which prevented greater gains in anemia control from being achieved.

Despite the presence of these major confounding factors, MICAH Malawi was still able to achieve a reduction in anemia prevalence in non-pregnant women. In the Comparison group however, no change was observed in non-pregnant women, and improvements seen in pregnant women in 2000 were lost by 2004. These findings indicate both the challenging context for anemia control in Malawi, and the fact that gains can still be made. A continued intensive effort is required to reduce anemia in Malawian women to a more acceptable level, particularly in the face of ongoing high HIV prevalence.

5.5.2. An Integrated Approach is Required to Address Anemia of Multi-Faceted Etiology

The association between several factors and women's hemoglobin, as presented in table 11, illustrates the importance of considering a variety of contributors to anemia when planning an effective intervention strategy. These include indirect contributors, such as women's education and household sanitation. MICAH Malawi implemented a comprehensive package of interventions for anemia prevention and control, as described earlier, and likely would not have seen positive results from only one or two isolated interventions. Conversely, achievement of greater coverage of some interventions, such as increased animal foods (e.g., small animals) and iron-fortified flour, would likely have increased the impact on anemia

---

[1] Van den Broek NK, White SA, Neilson JP. The relationship between asymptomatic Human Immunodeficiency Virus infection and the prevalence and severity of anemia in pregnant Malawian women. Am J Trop Med Hyg 1998;59(6):1004-1007.

prevalence. This is likely, as both Comparison and MICAH communities had similarly reduced levels of malaria and hookworm (as proxied by school children) in 2004, and so the main remaining contributor to anemia is likely to be dietary.

The association between presence of small animals in a household and women's hemoglobin is particularly noteworthy, indicating the critical importance of increased access to highly absorbable dietary iron. It is understood intuitively that improved dietary quality is the key to adequate iron intake and anemia reduction in populations with high levels of iron deficiency anemia and diets low in bioavailable iron. However there is a lack of published evidence of effective programming models that demonstrate a link between promotion of animal source foods and improved hemoglobin concentration in women. The MICAH Malawi results are therefore particularly valuable, and point to the legitimacy of investing in interventions that increase women's access to iron rich animal foods at the household level, accompanied by intensive nutrition education.

5.6. Conclusion

The MICAH program in Malawi invested considerably in anemia prevention and control using an integrated package of interventions designed to address the main contributors to anemia identified in the baseline survey (dietary iron intake, malaria and intestinal parasites). This approach proved to be successful in decreasing anemia prevalence in pregnant (1996 to 2000) and improving hemoglobin in non-pregnant (2000 to 2004) women of childbearing age. In particular, the emphasis on household rearing and consumption of small animals provides a programming model that may be suitable for replication in other similar rural African settings, as a means of increasing absorbable dietary iron intake.

The results achieved by MICAH Malawi are programmatically important, but anemia in both pregnant and non-pregnant women remains unacceptably high. It is likely that high HIV prevalence is a major contributor, set-backs from drought combined with inadequate dietary iron. While the success of the program demonstrates the validity of investment in anemia prevention and control in settings with high HIV prevalence, targets for anemia reduction need to take into account the impact of HIV. Although by 2004, MICAH Malawi achieved the goal of decreasing anemia among pregnant women by 19% over 8 years, and among non-pregnant women by 23% over 4 years, continued efforts need to be made to achieve the international goal of 30% reduction in anemia by 2010. Should Malawi also continue to face regular cycles of severe drought, achieving the international target will likely prove a significant challenge.

6.0. Summary of Case Studies

The MICAH program experience in Ghana and Malawi demonstrates that anemia prevention and control in women in developing countries is an achievable goal. However the approach and the expected results must take into account the local context.

In Ghana, iron deficiency was found to be the major cause of anemia in women, and an effective community-based IFA supplementation initiative was established, which led to dramatic reductions in anemia prevalence. Key success factors were the inclusion of all women of childbearing age as a target group for supplementation, and the use of community health volunteers to support the IFA distribution and provide appropriate health counseling messages regarding anemia and supplementation.

In Malawi anemia was found to have several contributors, including iron deficiency, malaria and intestinal parasites. The MICAH program addressed all of these with a comprehensive anemia prevention and control program. The interventions included distribution of small animals for household rearing and consumption through a revolving loan scheme, the pioneering of fortification technology for village mills, and public health measures to prevent malaria and hookworm infections. This comprehensive strategy was successful in reducing anemia prevalence in both pregnant and non-pregnant women, but the degree of improvement was lower than anticipated. Two major contextual factors that likely influenced this are high HIV prevalence and severe drought.

The following key lessons can be taken from the MICAH experience and applied in other developing countries:

- Analysis of the contributors to anemia and implementation of an integrated package of interventions is essential to designing an effective, context-specific anemia prevention and control program. Interventions to improve dietary iron intake need to be accompanied by public health control measures to address diseases such as malaria and hookworm which also contribute to anemia.
- In settings where iron deficiency anemia prevalence is in the severe public health range, IFA supplementation is necessary to improve hemoglobin levels. However at the same time the introduction of more sustainable strategies for the long-term maintenance of adequate iron status should be pursued. These strategies include fortification and dietary diversification.
- Community-based administration of anemia control interventions is critical to their success. Interventions should be integrated within existing structures and services, and implemented in partnership with relevant government ministries, community leaders and other agencies and partners as appropriate to the context.
- Dietary diversification, particularly the promotion of animal source foods, is a feasible strategy for sustainably improving intake and absorption of dietary iron and should be prioritized in anemia control programs.
- Monitoring the impact of program interventions is essential for improving the effectiveness of anemia prevention and control strategies. In addition to informing the program design and selection of interventions, MICAH survey results provided a valuable tool for advocacy to the national Ministries of Health for improved anemia control policies.

With the application of these programming principles, the international target for anemia reduction in women can be achieved. A renewed effort by the international health community towards this goal is required, but the MICAH experience demonstrates that with an integrated, comprehensive, context-specific program design, anemia in women can be effectively managed.

KEY POINTS

- Anemia is a prevalent international health problem which affects women and children commonly
- The consequences of anemia include fatigue, cognitive changes, decreased work productivity and increases morbidity and mortality of associated illnesses.
- Anemia is caused by iron deficiency, malaria, helminth infection, chronic diseases (ie., HIV/AIDS), reproductive disorders and genetics
- Programs to impact anemia like the MICAH program (Micronutrient and Health) in Ghana, Ethiopia and Malawi have been successful. The MICAH program is evidence based, comprehensive (with a multipronged intervention) and collaborative using partnerships with the health system and community.

REFERENCES

[1]   WHO/UNICEF/UNU. *Iron deficiency anaemia: assessment, prevention, and control.* Geneva: World Health Organization; 2001. (WHO/NHD/01.3)

[2]   WHO. *The prevalence of anaemia in women.* Geneva: World Health Organization;

[3]   1992. (WHO/MCH/MSM/92.2)

[4]   Brabin, B; Hakimi, M; Pelletier, D. An analysis of anemia and pregnancy-related maternal mortality. *J Nutr,* 2001 131, 604S-615S.

[5]   WHO/UNICEF/UNU. *Iron deficiency anaemia: assessment, prevention, and control.* Geneva: World Health Organization; 2001. (WHO/NHD/01.3)

[6]   *Resolution adopted by the General Assembly: S-27/2: A world fit for children.* United Nations General Assembly, 11 October 2002.

[7]   *We the children: end-decade review of the follow-up to the World Summit for Children: report of the Secretary-General.* United Nations General Assembly, 2001.

[8]   WHO/UNICEF/UNU. *Iron deficiency anaemia: assessment, prevention, and control.* Geneva: World Health Organization; 2001. (WHO/NHD/01.3)

[9]   WHO/UNICEF/UNU. *Iron deficiency anaemia: assessment, prevention, and control.* Geneva: World Health Organization; 2001. (WHO/NHD/01.3)

[10]   Galloway, R. *Anemia prevention and control: what works; part 1: program guidance.* USAID, World Bank, UNICEF, PAHO, FAO, MI, 2003.

[11]   ACC/SCN. *The 4th report on the world nutrition situation: Nutrition throughout the life cycle.* ACC/SCN in collaboration with the International Food Policy Research Institute. Geneva: ACC/SCN; 2000.

[12]   ACC/SCN. *The 4th report on the world nutrition situation: Nutrition throughout the life cycle.* ACC/SCN in collaboration with the International Food Policy Research Institute. Geneva: ACC/SCN.

[13]   Galloway R. *Anemia prevention and control: what works; part 1: program guidance.* USAID, World Bank, UNICEF, PAHO, FAO, MI, 2003.

[14]   WHO/UNICEF/UNU. *Iron deficiency anaemia: assessment, prevention, and control.* Geneva: World Health Organization; 2001. (WHO/NHD/01.3).

[15] FAO, WHO. *Human vitamin and mineral requirements*. Rome, Food and Agriculture Organization of the United Nations, 2001.

[16] Allen, LH; Ahluwalia, N. *Improving iron status through diet: The application of knowledge concerning dietary iron bioavailability in human populations*. Arlington VA: OMNI/John Snow, Inc.; 1997.

[17] Huddle, JM; Gibson, RS; Cullinan, TR. The impact of malaria infection and diet on the anaemia status of rural pregnant Malawian women. *Eur J Clin Nutr*, 1999 53(10), 792-801.

[18] Tatala, S; Svanberg, U; Mduma, B. Low dietary iron availability is a major cause of anemia: a nutrition survey in the Lindi District of Tanzania. *AJCN*, 1998 68, 171-8.

[19] Bhargava, A; Bouis, HE; Scrimshaw, NS. Dietary intakes and socioeconomic factors are associated with the hemoglobin concentration of Bangladeshi women. *J Nutr*, 2001 131, 758-764.

[20] WHO/UNICEF/UNU. *Iron deficiency anaemia: assessment, prevention, and control*. Geneva: World Health Organization; 2001. (WHO/NHD/01.3).

[21] WHO/UNICEF/UNU. *Iron deficiency anaemia: assessment, prevention, and control*. Geneva: World Health Organization; 2001. (WHO/NHD/01.3).

[22] Sloan, NL; Jordan, EA; Winikoff, B. Does iron supplementation make a difference? Arlington, VA: MotherCare Project, John Snow, Inc.; 1995. *(MotherCare Working Paper no. 15)*.

[23] Yip, R. Iron supplementation during pregnancy: is it effective? *Am J Clin Nutr*, 1996 63, 853-5.

[24] Yip, R. Iron supplementation during pregnancy: is it effective? *Am J Clin Nutr*, 1996 63, 853-5.

[25] WHO/UNICEF/UNU. *Iron deficiency anaemia: assessment, prevention, and control*. Geneva: World Health Organization; 2001. (WHO/NHD/01.3).

[26] Lotfi, M; Mannar, V; Merx, RJHM; Naber-van den Heuvel, P. Micronutrient fortification of foods: current practices, research and opportunities. Ottawa, *The Micronutrient Initiative*, 1996.

[27] World Bank. *Enriching lives: overcoming vitamin and mineral malnutrition in developing countries*. Washington DC: World Bank; 1994.

[28] Allen, LH; Ahluwalia, N. *Improving iron status through diet: The application of knowledge concerning dietary iron bioavailability in human populations*. Arlington VA: OMNI/John Snow, Inc.; 1997.

[29] van den Broek, NR; Letsky, EA. Etiology of anemia in pregnancy in south Malawi. *AJCN*, 2000 72(suppl), 247S-56S.

[30] Guyatt, HL; Snow, RW. The epidemiology and burden of Plasmodium falciparum-related anemia among pregnant women in sub-Saharan Africa. *Am J Trop Med Hyg*, 2001 Jan-Feb 64(1-2 suppl), 36-44.

[31] Verhoeff, FH; Brabin, BJ; Chimsuku, L; et al. Malaria in pregnancy and its consequences for the infant in rural Malawi. *Ann Trop Med Parasitol*, 1999 Dec 93 suppl 1, S25-33.

[32] Gillespie, S; Johnston, JL. Expert consultation on anemia determinants and interventions. Ottawa: *Micronutrient Initiative*; 1998.

[33] Shulman, CE; Dorman, EK. Importance and prevention of malaria in pregnancy. *Trans R Soc Trop Med Hyg*, 2003 Jan-Feb 97(1), 30-5.

[34] Verhoeff, FH; Brabin, BJ; Hart, CA; et al. Increased prevalence of malaria in HIV-infected pregnant women and its implications for malaria control. *Trop Med Int Health*, 1999 Jan 4(1), 5-12.

[35] Shulman, CE; Dorman, EK; Cutts, F; et al. Intermittent sulphadoxine-pyrimethamine to prevent severe anaemia secondary to malaria in pregnancy: a randomized placebo-controlled trial. *Lancet*, 1999 Feb 20 353(9153), 632-6.

[36] Rogerson, SJ; Chaluluka, E; Kanjala, M; et al. Intermittent sulfadoxine-pyrimethamine in pregnancy: effectiveness against malaria morbidity in Blantyre, Malawi, in 1997-99. *Trans R Soc Trop Med Hyg*, 2000 Sep-Oct 94(5), 549-53.

[37] Marchant, T; Schellenberg, JA; Edgar, T; et al. Socially marketed insecticide-treated nets improve malaria and anaemia in pregnancy in southern Tanzania. *Trop Med Int Health*, 2002 Feb 7(2), 149-58.

[38] *Roll Back Malaria Partnership*. Global strategic plan, 2005-2015. Geneva, RBM Partnership Secretariat, 2005.

[39] Stoltzfus, RJ; Dreyfuss, ML; Chwaya, HM; Albonico, M. Hookworm control as a strategy to prevent iron deficiency. *Nutr Rev*, 1997 Jun 55(6), 223-32.

[40] Dreyfuss, ML; Stoltzfus, RJ; Shrestha, JB; et al. Hookworms, malaria and vitamin A deficiency contribute to anemia and iron deficiency among pregnant women in the plains of Nepal. *J Nutr*, 2000 130, 2527-2536.

[41] World Health Organization. *Report of the WHO Consultation on hookworm infection and anaemia in girls and women*. Geneva: WHO; 1994. (WHO/CTD/SIP/96.1).

[42] Galloway, R. *Anemia prevention and control: what works; part 1: program guidance.* USAID, World Bank, UNICEF, PAHO, FAO, MI, 2003.

[43] Piwoz, EG; Preble, EA. HIV/AIDS and nutrition: A review of the literature and recommendations for nutritional care and support in sub-Saharan Africa. Washington DC:*Support for Analysis and Research in Africa/AED project*, 2000.

[44] Van den Broek, NR; White, SA; Neilson, JP. The relationship between asymptomatic Human Immunodeficiency Virus infection and the prevalence and severity of anemia in pregnant Malawian women. *Am J Trop Med Hyg*, 1998 59(6), 1004-1007.

[45] Antelman, G; Msamanga, GI; Spiegelman, D; et al. Nutritional factors and infectious disease contribute to anemia among pregnant women with Human Immunodeficiency Virus in Tanzania. *J Nutr*, 2000 130, 1950-1957.

[46] Galloway, R. *Anemia prevention and control: what works; part 1: program guidance.* USAID, World Bank, UNICEF, PAHO, FAO, MI, 2003.

[47] Galloway, R. *Anemia prevention and control: what works; part 1: program guidance.* USAID, World Bank, UNICEF, PAHO, FAO, MI, 2003.

[48] Massawe, SN. Anaemia in women of reproductive age in Tanzania. A study in Dar-es-Salaam. Acta Universitatis Upsaliensis. *Comprehensive Summaries of Uppsala Dissertations from the Faculty of Medicine* 1151. Uppsala, 2002.

[49] Tatala, S; Svanberg, U; Mduma, B. Low dietary iron availability is a major cause of anemia: a nutrition survey in the Lindi District of Tanzania. *AJCN*, 1998 68, 171-8.

[50] Dreyfuss, ML; Stoltzfus, RJ; Shrestha, JB; et al. Hookworms, malaria and vitamin A deficiency contribute to anemia and iron deficiency among pregnant women in the plains of Nepal. *J Nutr*, 2000 130, 2527-2536.

[51] Haas, JD; Brownlie, T IV. Iron deficiency and reduced work capacity: a critical review of the research to determine a causal relationship. *J Nutr*, 2001 131, 676S-690S.

[52] WHO/UNICEF/UNU. *Iron deficiency anaemia: assessment, prevention, and control.* Geneva: World Health Organization; 2001. (WHO/NHD/01.3).

[53] Levin, H. A benefit-cost analysis of nutritional interventions for anemia reduction. *Population, Health and Nutrition Department Technical Note 85-12.* Washington DC: World Bank; 1985.

[54] Grantham-McGregor, S; Ani, C. A review of studies on the effect of iron deficiency on cognitive development in children. *J Nutr,* 2001 131, 649S-668S.

[55] Ross, J; Horton, S. Economic consequences of iron deficiency. Ottawa*: Micronutrient Initiative;* 1998.

[56] Brabin, BJ; Hakimi, M; Pelletier, D. An analysis of anemia and pregnancy-related maternal mortality. *J Nutr,* 2001 131, 604S-615S.

[57] Rush, D. Nutrition and maternal mortality. *Am J Clin Nutr,* 2000 72(suppl), 212S-40S.

[58] Vitamin and mineral deficiency: A global progress report. *The Micronutrient Initiative,* UNICEF, 2003.

[59] UN SCN. *Nutrition for Improved Development Outcomes: 5th Report on the World Nutrition Situation.* Geneva: 2004.

[60] Wagstaff, A; Claeson, M. *The Millennium Development Goals for health: rising to the challenges.* Washington: The World Bank; 2004.

[61] Allen, LH. Anemia and iron deficiency: effects on pregnancy outcome. *Am J Clin Nutr,* 2000 71(suppl), 1280S-4S.

[62] Ashworth, A. Effects of intrauterine growth retardation on mortality and morbidity in infants and young children. *Eur J Clin Nutr,* 1998 52(S1), 34-42.

[63] De Pee, S; Bloem, MW; Sari, M; et al. The high prevalence of low hemoglobin concentration among Indonesian infants aged 3-5 months is related to maternal anemia. *J Nutr,* 2002 132(8), 2215-21.

[64] Yip, R. Significance of an abnormally low or high hemoglobin concentration during pregnancy: special consideration of iron nutrition. *Am J Clin Nutr,* 2000 72(suppl), 272S-9S.

[65] Yip, R. Iron supplementation during pregnancy: is it effective? *Am J Clin Nutr,* 1996 63, 853-5.

[66] Galloway, R; Dusch, E; Elder, L; et al. Women's perceptions of iron deficiency and anemia prevention and control in eight developing countries. *Soc Sci Med,* 2002 Aug 55(4), 529-44.

[67] Trowbridge, F. Prevention and control of iron deficiency: priorities and action steps. *J Nutr,* 2002 132, 880S-882S.

[68] Joint statement by the World Health Organization and the United Nations Children's Fund. *Focusing on anemia: towards an integrated approach for effective anaemia control.* Geneva: WHO; 2004.

[69] Winichagoon, P. Prevention and control of anemia: Thailand experiences. J Nutr, 2002 132, 862S-866S.

[70] Egypt's Adolescent Anemia Prevention Program: A report on program development, pilot efforts and lessons learned. *Ministry of Health and Population and Health Insurance Organization.*

[71] *MotherCare. Malawi maternal anemia program 1995-1998. Technical Working Paper #10.* Arlington, Va.: MotherCare/John Snow, Inc., project, 2000.

[72] Gleason, GR; Sharmanov, T. Anemia prevention and control in four Central Asian republics and Kazakhstan. *J Nutr,* 2002 132, 867S-870S.

[73] UNAIDS data: *http://www.unaids.org/en/Regions_Countries/Countries/ghana.asp.*

[74] *MICAH Ghana Baseline Survey Report.* World Vision, 1997.

[75] *MICAH Ghana. Final Survey Report,* 2006. World Vision Canada, 1 World Drive, Mississauga, Ontario.

[76] Beaton, GH; McCabe, GP. Efficacy of intermittent iron supplementation in the control of iron deficiency anemia in developing countries. *The Micronutrient Initiative,* Ottawa, 1999.

[77] Bothwell, TH. Iron requirements in pregnancy and strategies to meet them. *Am J Clin Nutr, 2000* 72(suppl), 257S-64S.

[78] *MICAH Ghana Final Survey Report.* World Vision, 2006.

[79] Viteri, FE; Berger, J. Importance of pre-pregnancy and pregnancy iron status: can long-term weekly preventive iron and folic acid supplementation achieve desirable and safe status? *Nutr Rev,* 2005 Dec 63(12 Pt 2):S65-76.

[80] Allen, LH. Iron supplements: scientific issues concerning efficacy and implications for research and programs. *J Nutr,* 2002 132, 813S-819S.

[81] Berger, J; Thanh, HT; Cavalli-Sforza, T; et al. Community mobilization and social marketing to promote weekly iron-folic acid supplementation in women of reproductive age in Vietnam: impact on anemia and iron status. *Nutr Rev,* 2005 Dec 63(12 Pt 2), S95-108.

[82] Bothwell, TH. Iron requirements in pregnancy and strategies to meet them. *Am J Clin Nutr, 2000* 72(suppl), 257S-64S.

[83] Yip, R. Iron supplementation during pregnancy: is it effective? *Am J Clin Nutr,* 1996 63, 853-5.

[84] Yip, R. Iron supplementation: country level experiences and lessons learned. *J Nutr,* 2002 132, 859S-861S.

[85] Jus'at, I; Achadi, EL; Galloway, R; et al. Reaching young Indonesian women through marriage registries: an innovative approach for anemia control. *J Nutr,* 2000 130, 456S-458S.

[86] UNAIDS data: www.unaids.org/en/Regions_Countries/Countries/malawi.asp.

[87] Van den Broek, NK; White, SA; Neilson, JP. The relationship between asymptomatic Human Immunodeficiency Virus infection and the prevalence and severity of anemia in pregnant Malawian women. *Am J Trop Med Hyg,* 1998 59(6), 1004-1007.

[88] *MICAH Malawi Final Survey Report.* World Vision, 2006.

[89] Habicht, JP; Victora, CG; Vaughan, JP. Evaluation designs for adequacy, plausibility and probability of public health programme performance and impact. *Int J Epid,* 1999 28, 10-18.

In: Women's Health in the Majority World: Issues and Initiatives   ISBN1-1-60021-493-2
Eds: L. Elit and J. Chamberlain Froese, pp. 109-131   © 2007 Nova Science Publishers, Inc.

Chapter 6

EXPLORING FAIRNESS IN HEALTH CARE REFORM[*]

Rebecca J. Cook

Faculty of Law, University of Toronto, Canada and
Department of Constitutional Law and Philosophy of Law,
University of the Free State, South Africa

ABSTRACT

This article considers the increasing challenge of the fair allocation of scarce public health care resources by focusing on services for women and girls. It considers different ways of thinking about fairness in health care reform, the role of courts in promoting fairness, and the use of affirmative action measures to remedy health disparities. The health of individuals and populations is shown to be affected by clinical services, the organization and functioning of health systems, and underlying socio-economic determinants. Different theories of justice are addressed that affect assessments of fairness, considering availability, accessibility, acceptability of and accountability for services. The transition in judicial dispositions is traced, from deference to governmental resource allocation decisions to evidence-based scrutiny of governmental observance of constitutional and human rights legal obligations. The appropriate use of affirmative action measures to improve equality in health status is explored, given the increasingly unacceptable disparities in health among subgroups of women within countries.

1. INTRODUCTION

Fairness in health care reform, both within a country and among countries, is becoming an increasingly pressing national and international challenge. The reasons are many. They include:

---

[*]This article is an adaptation of an Inaugral lecture delivered by Professor R. Cook in acceptance of her appointment as Professor Extraordinarius in the Department of Constitutional law and Philosophy of law, University of the Free State. Originally published in the Journal for Judicial science 29(3):1-27 (2004). Permission for reprint given by author and journal.

- Rising costs and expectations of health care, and related reforms that may cause public rationing of scarce health resources,
- The growing intolerance of health disparities and unfair health outcomes among groups, whether disparities are due to unequal availability of or unequal access to, services.

Examples of health disparities and unfair health outcomes include preventable premature death due to differential prevalence rates of HIV/AIDS among different income groups, differential rates of unwanted pregnancy among different age groups, and differential rates of maternal mortality and morbidity between northern and southern countries. The underlying conditions necessary for health, such as safe drinking water, sanitation, adequate income, education and housing, and empowerment of communities marginalized by sex, race, and age, also vary within and among countries. In addition to these explanations of growing attention to fairness in health care reform, is a more generalized reason of an informed and engaged citizenry that seeks to protect health as a fundamental value, and is increasingly requiring government to ensure reasonable availability of and access to health services.

Where democratic governments are not providing such services, they risk being voted out of office or being held accountable for fair and effective provision through court challenges using constitutional and human rights principles. In some countries, such as Canada, where there is no explicit constitutional protection of health [1] access to health care is viewed as part and parcel of the right of nondiscrimination [2] and, for example, the right to security of the person [3]. In other countries, such as South Africa, where there is specific constitutional protection of the right to health care [4], this right is being interpreted to require fair access to health care [5].

There are many governmental health care reform initiatives [6], including moves toward decentralization, emphasis on cost recovery, and an expanded role for the private sector. Each one of these initiatives justifies an article in itself. This article will explore fairness in health services, especially as it impacts on women and girls, by looking at three matters:

- Different ways of thinking about fairness in health care reform,
- The role of the courts in promoting fairness in health resource allocation, and
- The use of affirmative action to promote equality in health.

---

[1] The Canadian Charter of Rights and Freedoms, part I of the Constitution Act, 1982, being Schedule B to the Canada Act 1982 (U.K.), 1982, chapter 11.

[2] *Eldridge v British Columbia (Attorney General)* (1977), 151 D.L.R. (4th) 577 (The Supreme Court of Canada decided that failure to provide funding for sign language interpretation that would equip hearing-impaired patients to communicate with health services providers in the same way that unimpaired patients can, constitutes discrimination in violation of Section 15(1) of the Canadian Charter of Rights and Freedoms).

[3] *R v Morgentaler* (1988) 44 DLR (4th) 385 (The Supreme Court of Canada held that the restrictions of the criminal abortion law violated a women's right to security of the person protected by Section 7 of the Canadian Charter of Rights and Freedoms).

[4] South African Constitution, sections 27(1)(a), 28(1)(b) and (c)

[5] *Minister of Health v Treatment Action Campaign* (No 2) 2002 (5) SA 721. The Constitutional Court of South Africa held that reasonable provision of treatment to pregnant women with HIV/AIDS is required by the right to health care services of the South African Constitution.

[6] See Canada. Commission on the Future of Health Care in Canada 2002.

The thesis is that courts have a significant role to play in the dynamics of health care reform, and remedying inequities that result from stagnation or misguided reforms in allocation of scarce health resources.

Health is affected by:

- clinical services,
- health systems, and
- the underlying socio-economic conditions and other determinants of health [7].

Medicine focuses on improving the health of individuals in the context of clinical services to treat physical and to a lesser extent mental illness. Health systems go beyond clinical services to determine how the health of populations can be maximized. Health systems use epidemiological and health systems research to plan and implement health interventions that emphasize prevention of diseases and promotion of health. Social science research has underscored the importance of underlying conditions and determinants, and the importance of socio-economic, gender and racial factors in affecting health outcomes.

Courts continue to play a significant role in regulating the delivery of clinical services, by ensuring respect for patient autonomy [8] and, for example, patient confidentiality [9]. Recent efforts to reform health care are now requiring courts to scrutinize the fairness of decisions at health system levels; that is, of choice of ministries of health, in allocating scarce health resources. Just as courts have developed an important body of jurisprudence and norms regulating the delivery of clinical care, so too is their role significant in developing norms and standards at the health systems levels, especially in the fairness of allocating scarce health resources. This article concentrates on fairness in structuring and funding governmental health systems.

2. WAYS OF THINKING ABOUT FAIRNESS IN HEALTH CARE REFORM

Fairness in health care reform is likely to be contentious because of competing interests. There are many different ways of thinking about fairness [10]. One approach to fairness explains that fairness is a health care system requires, at a minimum, equity in health outcomes, reasonable availability of health care, efficiency in management of services, patient autonomy, and accountability [11].

Underlying any approach to fairness in health resource allocation are theories of justice, which include compensatory justice, distributive justice, utilitarian and liberal theories of justice [12]. Compensatory justice justifies the use of measures that compensate particular groups for historical wrongs they have suffered. When this rationale is applied, proof of past discrimination is usually necessary, to ensure that measures achieve correction only to the

---

[7] Cook et al 2003;218-221, 256-259
[8] *Reibl v Hughes* (1980), 114 D.L.R. (3d) 1 (Supreme Court of Canada)
[9] *W v Egdell* [1990] 1 All E.R. 835 (English Court of Appeal).
[10] Dahlgren and Whitehead 1991.
[11] Daniels et al 2000a; Daniels et al 2002; Daniels et al 1996; Daniels et al 2000b.
[12] Beauchamp and Childress 2001:230-235; Raday 2003:35-44

extent of those past wrongs. Debates often center on the extent of the discriminatory harm, and the nature of the proof that is necessary to show the harm.

Compensatory justice may have little to offer in the health field, since mandating fair treatment for those who have suffered historical wrongs will not be compensation for them, but only the fair enforcement of nondiscriminatory health policies to which they are properly entitled. That is, the required measures do not provide any special advantage, but rather enforcement of measures equal to those that comparable individuals and groups have been accustomed to enjoy.

In contrast to compensatory justice that focuses on making up for unfair past treatment, distributive justice rationale is prospective in focus. It may be employed to justify future equitable availability of health resources to subgroups at abnormally high levels of risk. For instance, affirmative action might be justified to develop early diagnosis of cervical cancer and treatment programs for subgroups of women at high risk, until such time as their survival rate is the same as that of the general population. In other words, courts can require the temporary allocation of scarce resources in order to reduce present or anticipated exceptional need.

A utilitarian rational may be employed to introduce measures to improve the welfare and capacities of the female half of society in order to increase overall social satisfaction, and productivity. This rationale might justify programs to promote equality in availability of services to ensure that women's distinctive health needs are satisfied, such as maternity care.

A liberal theory of justice justifies empowerment of women as autonomous, rational agents to determine their own clinical care, and remove barriers, such as husbands' authorization requirements, to access to care. Liberal theories can be criticized for overemphasizing abstract notions of autonomy, and not taking sufficient account of women's contexts and the underlying determinants of health such as how societies structure women's reproductive and productive roles in ways that disadvantage their access to services.

These and other theories of social justice are examined from different feminist perspectives to determine the extent to which they accommodate women's needs and interests [13]. Relevant to theories of justice and considerations of fairness within health care systems is the work of many disciplines, including the contributions of philosophy [14] political science [15], public health and epidemiology [16], law [17] and, for example, sociology and health systems [18]

This article will draw on different disciplines and theories of justice, and use the framework of the Right to the Highest Attainable Standard of Health, protected by the International Covenant on Economic, Social and Cultural Rights (the Economic Covenant)[19]. The Covenant's monitoring body, the Committee on Economic, Social and Cultural Rights (the Economic Committee) has developed a General Comment on the Right to the Highest Attainable Standard of Health [20].

---

[13] Lacey 2003;13-55

[14] Daniels et al 2000a

[15] Tuohy 1999.

[16] Braveman and Gruskin 2003a:583; Braveman 2003:181-192; Braveman and Gruskin 2003b:254-258

[17] Flood 2000

[18] Van Rensburg 2004; Doyal 2000:931-939

[19] Article 12, International Covenant on Economic, Social and Cultural Rights, 16Dec. 1966, 993 UNTS 3, entered into force 3Jan1976

[20] Committee on Economic, Social and Cultural Right, General Comment 14: The right to the highest attainable standard of health, CESCR, General Comment 14, UN ESCOR 2000, UN Doc. E/C. 12/2000/4, 11August2000

This Comment on the Right to Health provides guidance to the Covenant's member countries in reporting to the Economic Committee on what they have done to protect this right to satisfy the criteria of what are described as the four A's. These criteria require that health services are: available, accessible, acceptable, and where they are not, to ensure that government is accountable to remedy deficiencies in availability, accessibility or acceptability in health care delivery.

This General Comment explains that 'States parties have a core obligation to ensure the satisfaction of, at the very least, minimum essential levels of each of the rights enunciated in the Covenant, including essential primary health care' [21]. It needs to be read in conjunction with General comment on the Nature of States parties Obligations under Article 2 (1) of the Covenant, with reads in part:

A State party in which any significant number of individuals is deprived of ...essential primary health care ...is, prima facie, failing to discharge its obligations under the Covenant. If the Covenant were to be read in such a way as not to establish such a minimum core obligation, it would be largely deprived of its raison d'etre. By the same token, it must be noted that any assessment as to whether a State has discharged its minimum core obligations must also take account of resource constraints applying within the country concerned. Article 2(1) obligates each Stage party to take the necessary steps 'to the maximum of its available resources'. In order for a State party to be able to attribute its failure to meet at least its minimum core obligations to a lack of available resource it must demonstrate that every effort has been made to use all resources that are at its disposition in an effort to satisfy, as a matter of priority, those minimum obligations [22].

The General Comment of the Right to Health, read together with the General Comment on State Obligations, require that states parties ensure that a minimum core of primary health care is available, accessible and acceptable.

2.1. Availability

The General Comment on the Right to Health explains that the minimum core includes the obligation of states to ensure the right of access to health facilities, goods and services on a nondiscriminatory basis, especially for vulnerable or marginalized groups, and the provision of essential drugs as determined by the World Health Organization have to be available in sufficient quantity. The precise nature of the facilities, goods and services will vary depending on numerous factors. They include the underlying determinants of health, such as safe drinking water and adequate sanitation facilities [23]. Most significantly, these minimum core rights are non-derogable: 'a State party cannot, under any circumstances whatsoever, justify its non-compliance with the core obligations' [24].

---

[21] General Comment 14, par 43; Chapman 2002;185-215
[22] Committee on Economic, Social and Cultural Rights, General Comment 3, The nature of State Parties Obligations (article 2(1)), UN Doc. E/1991/23 (1990), par 10.
[23] General Comment 14, par 43.
[24] General Comment 14, par 47

In terms of women's health, one needs to ask how health care reform ensures availability of services specific to their health needs, and whether services are delivered in ways that are responsive to women's needs. One commentator has explained that:

> A women's health needs approach is concerned with the implications for women of differences in the epidemiological profile between the sexes. This approach highlights the specific health needs of women and girls as a consequence particularly (although not exclusively) of the biology of reproduction [25].

The same commentator explains that two broad strands flow from this approach.

One stresses the need to provide specific, women focused health care interventions as a basic right in order to address the imbalance of need. The rights approach to women's health needs is underscored by the right to sexual non-discrimination. This right requires that like cases be treated alike and different cases be treated according to their differences. In the context of women's health, the right to non-discrimination requires that societies treat different biological interests, such as in pregnancy and childbirth, in ways that reasonably accommodate those interests. The Convention on the Elimination of All Forms of Discrimination against Women (the Women's Convention) requires member states to ensure equality by protecting women's distinct interests in health [26].

The other approach emphasizes the cost effectiveness of interventions which focus on women and girls (particularly reproductive health interventions), both in comparison to other types of interventions and as a means to improve the health of those dependent on women's care, namely infants and children [27]. The cost effectiveness rational is further reinforced by a wider theme of investing in women's health, to reduce the overall economic burden in communities of disease and poverty.

Whether a rights justification to promote women's health or a cost effectiveness rationale is employed, accommodating women's health needs requires provisions of services specific to their health needs, such as to prevent unwanted pregnancy, to treat the consequences of unwanted pregnancy, and to secure safe pregnancy, childbirth and neonatal care, and for example, early diagnosis and treatment of cervical cancer. Moreover, serving women's health needs requires that governments address the underlying conditions that lead to ill-health, such as societal tolerance of violence against women and abusive sexual practices.

2.2. Accessibility

The Economic Committee's General Comment requires that health facilities, goods and services have to be accessible to everyone. Accessibility has interrelated dimensions, such as:

- Nondiscrimination,
- Physical accessibility, and

---

[25] Standing 1997:1-18

[26] Article 12, Convention on the Elimination of All Forms of Discrimination against Women, 18Dec. 1979, GA Res. 34/180, UNGAOR, 34th Sess, Supp. No. 46 at 193, of Discrimination against Women, General Recommendation 24, women and health in HRI/Gen/1/Rev.4 (2000)

[27] Standing 1997:1-2

-    Affordability [28].

If health care facilities, personnel and resources are to be accessible, governments must do more than simply provide them as bulk services. Accessibility requires that the delivery and administration of health care is organized in a fair, nondiscriminatory manner, with special attention to the most vulnerable and marginalized. The enumerated grounds of discrimination are open ended, and include race, sex sexual orientation, physical and mental disability and health status [29].

Administration of health care has to respond to the medical, as well as, psychological, social and economic needs of the health care system users [30]. Research has provided insights into how constructions of gender 'produce vulnerability to ill health or disadvantage within health care systems and particularly the conditions which promote inequality between the sexes in relation to access and utilization of services' [31].

2.3. Acceptability

The General Comment requires that all health facilities, goods and services must be respectful of medical ethics, and be culturally appropriate [32]. That is, they must be respectful of marginalized groups, and sensitive to gender and life cycle requirements, as well as being designed to respect confidentiality. A subset of acceptability is the requirement that services be 'scientifically and medically appropriate and of good quality' [33].

Services are not acceptable when they lack quality, fail to protect free and informed decision making and, for example, neglect to respect confidentiality. Studies show, for instance, that where confidentiality is not respected, adolescent girls are deterred from seeking reproductive and related health care [34]. Where services, such for treatment for cervical cancer or sexually transmitted diseases, are not delivered in respectful, non-stigmatizing ways, women are deterred from seeking early diagnosis and treatment [35].

2.4. Accountability

All sectors of society, including those marginalized by sex, age, disability, race, and or poverty, must be able to hold the health system accountable for lack of availability, accessibility and acceptability of services, and more widely their obligations regarding the right to the highest attainable standard of health [36]. The General Comment on health explains that victims of violations should have 'access to effective judicial or other appropriate

---

[28] General Comment 14, par 12.
[29] General Comment 14, par 18.
[30] Health Canada 2001.
[31] Standing 1997:2.
[32] General Comment 14,par 12.
[33] General Comment 14, par 12.
[34] Ford et al 1997:1029-34.
[35] Gomez-Jauregui et al 2004.
[36] General Comment 14, pars 57-58; N. Daniels et al 2000a.

remedies ...' [37] This is a provision to which the courts in many countries are responding, by becoming willing to provide remedies to ensure fairness in availability of and access to public health services.

Claimants before courts may draw on the results of health systems studies to show disparities, and governments responding to judicial demands for effective remedies of unfair policies may similarly turn to such studies, to show their reformed compliance with required standards.

An emerging issue for governments to show compliance with standards and for those challenging governmental decisions is to identify approaches that can be taken to determine whether governments have complied with their human rights obligations. Two approaches are through human rights needs assessments, and gender-based analysis.

- Human rights needs assessments are designed to determine whether health systems are complying with their obligations to ensure that needed services are available, accessible and acceptable [38].
- Gender-based analysis is designed to determine whether and how women's health needs are accommodated, and to identify opportunities to improve services on which women's health depends [39].

These approaches are not mutually exclusive, and are perhaps best explored in combination.

A key question in both approaches is the choice of indicators to assess availability, accessibility and acceptability of health care services. The UN Special Rapporteur on the Right to Health has suggested that three broad categories of indicators might be useful in assessing state compliance with the right to health, namely:

- structural indicators,
- process indicators and
- outcomes indicators [40].

Structural indicators, which include health policy indicators, 'address whether or not key structures, systems and mechanisms that are considered necessary for, or conducive to, the realization of the right to health are in place' [41].

Structural indicators address laws and policies, as well as the outcomes of these policies. They may be examined by such question, for examples, as:

- Does the state constitutionalize the right to health?
- Has the government adopted a national strategy and plan of action to reduce maternal mortality?

---

[37] General Comment 14, par 59.

[38] Gostin and Lazzarini 1997;57-67.

[39] Health Canada 2003.

[40] commission on Human Rights, Note by the Secretary General: Interim Report of the Special rapporteur of the Commission on Human Rights on the Right of Everyone to the Enjoyment of the Highest Attainable Standard of Physical and mental health, Mr. Paul Hunt, A/58/427, 10Oct2003, para. 15.

[41] Interim Report of Special Rapporteur, par 19.

- Does the government have an Essential Medicines List?
- Which medicines are free of charge at primary public health facilities; (including) HIV/AIDS-related medicines, and free medicines for under fives/pregnant women/elderly/all who cannot afford them? [42]

Structural indicators might also explore the extent to which health systems produce or exacerbate vulnerabilities of groups marginalized by sex, race or, for example, age that contribute to their health disadvantage or disease burden. For example, the socio-cultural constructions of gender might usefully be examined to determine how they inhibit or accommodate women's health needs and access to services.

Process indicators, which include health service indicators, 'provide information on the processes by which a health policy is implemented. They measure the degree to which activities that are necessary to attain certain health objectives are fulfilled, and the progress of those activities over time. They monitor, as it were, effort, not outcome[43]. Examples of process indicators include:

- ...number of facilities with functioning basic essential obstetric care per 500,000 population.
- percentage of people with advanced HIV infection receiving antiretroviral combination therapy [44].

Outcome indicators, which include health status indicators, 'measure the results achieved by health-related policies. They show the 'facts' about people's health, such as maternal mortality, prevalence of HIV, prevalence of rape...'[45]

These indicators assist in thinking about fairness, and have strengths and weaknesses [46]. A difficulty with indicators is that it might be difficult to determine how services should accommodate different reproductive functions of the sexes and how the different hormonal and genetic constitution of the sexes affects non-reproductive facets of health, such as in the different incidence of disabilities and reactions to medical interventions. In addition to the hormonal and genetic factors, there are underlying socio-economic conditions that affect health outcomes. Consequently, health outcomes indicators are useful but not conclusive when determining allocations of scarce health resources. In order to address differential health outcomes, health ministries will have to address hormonal and genetic factors and other militating factors such as underlying socio-economic conditions. Indicators will develop over time as understandings of the causes and consequences of health disparities evolve through improved dialogue among the different disciplines.

---

[42] Interim Report of Special Rapporteur 2003, para 20.
[43] Interim Report of Special Rapporteur 2003, para 26.
[44] Interim Report of Special Rapporteur 2003, para 27.
[45] Interim Report of Special Rapporteur 2003, par 28.
[46] Cook et al 2003:225-228.

3. The Role of Courts in Promoting Fairness in Health Resource Allocation

National courts spanning the globe, from Australia to Venezuela, from South Africa to Canada, are now acting as forums for public deliberation on health care rationing. International human rights tribunals and committees are also considering questions of fair access to health care. Whether before national or international courts, governments are now required to justify the choices they have made in allocating public resources, according to human rights principles. Governments have to explain the criteria that underpin their decisions, and satisfy the courts that they have considered all interests, but only relevant interests. Courts are requiring greater transparency in decision-making, whether it be in scientific review, or in fairness in the process of review. Generally in the area of allocation of health care resources, courts are moving from a mode of deference to the executive branch of government, to a mode of deliberation [47].

Common complaints against government allocation decisions concern those of discrimination in access to care, or denied or delayed access. The grounds on which discrimination claims are made include sex [48], race [49], health status or disability [50], marital status [51], and sexual orientation [52]. Where there is no discrimination in access to care, courts are being asked to decide whether denial of basic health care [53], is a form of inhuman or degrading treatment, or whether it infringes rights to life [54] or security [55], or offends

---

[47] Syrett 2004;190-198.

[48] New Mexico Right to Choose/NARAL v William Johnson, Secretary of the New Mexico Human Services Department, 126 N.M. 788, 792 (1999) Supreme Court of New Mexico (the state's prohibition of funding for medically necessary abortions denies Medicaid-eligible women equality under the law because it does not apply the same standard of medical necessity to men and women).

[49] Linton v Tenn. Community Health and Environmental, 779 F. Supp. 925, affirmed 923 F. 2d 855 (6th Cir. 1981) (bed certifications polices with adverse disparate impact on racial and ethnic minorities held discriminatory and in violation of title VI of the Civil Rights Act and the Medicaid statute).

[50] Eldridge v British Columbia (Attorney General) (1977), 151 D.L.R. (4th) 577. (The Supreme Court of Canada decided that failure to provide funding for sign language interpretation that would equip hearing-impaired patients to communicate with health services provides in the same way that unimpaired patients can constitute discrimination in violation of the Canadian Charter on Rights and Freedoms); Auton (Guardian ad Litem of) v British Columbia (Attorney General) (2002) 220 D.L.R. (4th) 411 (B.C.C.A.) (The British Columbia Court of Appear upheld British Columbia Supreme Court's decision in finding that governmental failure to provide services for autistic children constituted discrimination on grounds of disability in violation of the Canadian Charter of Rights and Freedoms, and could not be said to be reasonable justifiable.) An appeal is pending before the Canadian Supreme Court; Cameron v Nova Scotia Attorney General (1999) D.L.R. (4th) 611 (The Nova Scotia Court of Apeal Decided that Nova Scotia's refusal to fund infertility services, while discriminatory, was justified due to costs and lack of proven effectiveness.)

[51] *McBain v Victoria* (2000) 3 Commonwealth Human Rights law 153 (denying an unmarried woman artificial insemination violates her right to nondiscrimination on the ground of marital statu) Federal Court of Appeal or Australia.

[52] *Korn v Potter* (1996) 134 DLR (4th) 437 (denying a lesbian woman artificial insemination is a violation of her right to nondiscrimination on the ground of sexual orientation) Supreme Court of British Columbia.

[53] Case 7615 (Brazil) (1985), Inter-Am. Comm. H.R. Rex. No. 12/85, Annual Report of the Inter-American Commission on Human Rights, 1984-1985. (The Commission held Brazil responsible for failure to take effective measures to preserve health of the Yanomami Indians pursuant to Article XI of the American Declaration of the Rights and Duties of Man).

[54] *X v United Kingdon* (1978), Eur. Comm. H.R. Application No 7154, Decision 12 July 1978, European Commission of Human Right, Decision and Reports 14:31-35, June 1979. (U.K. had taken appropriate measures to prevent death from vaccination but had appropriate measures not been taken, the state would have been in breach of its duty to safeguard life under Article 2 of the European Convention on Human Rights).

complainants' right to health care [56]. This has arisen in such areas as fair access to emergency care [57], palliative care [58], treatment for HIV/AIDS[59], kidney failure [60] and care for prisoners [61].

Where judicial determination on the merits of cases is pending, courts will generally apply the precautionary principle to prevent the risk of harm beyond the courts' means of subsequent remedy. The precautionary principle provides that, even in the absence of scientific evidence of cause and effect relationships, precaution should be taken to preserve the status quo in case the effects of change would prove disastrous to the important interests at stake. Courts are applying the precautionary principle to require governments to provide interim health care pending their judicial decisions [62].

3.1. Deference

Historically, barriers to private individuals and institutions bringing actions in courts have shielded governmental policies from judicial scrutiny. Barriers have included legal doctrines of state immunity from proceedings brought against governments in their national courts. Government bureaucracies have been unaccustomed to having to justify their policies before

---

[55] *R. V Morgentaler* (1988) 44 DLR (4th) 385 (the restrictions of the criminal abortion law violated a woman's right to security of the person under the Canadian Charter of Rights and Freedoms).

[56] *Treatment Action Campaign;* Cruz *Bermudez, et al. v Ministerio de Sanidad y Asistencia Social (MSAS),* Case No. 15789, 1999 (Pursuant to the rights to life and health, the Venezuelan Supreme Court required the Ministry of Health to probide the medicines prescribed to all HIV positive Venezuelans by government doctors, cover the cost of HIV blood tests in order for patients to obtain the necessary anti-retroviral treatments and treatments for opportunistic infections, develop the policies and programs necessary for treatment of affected patients, and make the reallocation of the budget necessary to carry out the decision of the Court (Articles 58, 76, the 1961 Venezuelan Constitution).

[57] *Paschim Banga Khet Mazdoor Samity v State of West Bengal* (1996) 4 SCC 37; (1996) 3SCJ 25, digested in (1998) 2 Commonwealth Human Rights Law Digest 109. (The Supreme Court of India held that the right to life protected by Article 21 of the Indian Constitution was breached when various government hospitals denied a complainant emergency treatment for serious head injuries.).

[58] *D v United Kingdom* (1997), Eur. Ct. H. R. 24 E.H.R.R. 423. (The European Court of Human Rights held that the U.K. could not deport a convicted drug trafficker, who was at a very advanced stage of terminal and incurable AIDS, to his native country where he would not receive appropriate care, would constitute inhuman treatment contrary to Article 3 of the European Convention on Human Rights.).

[59] Treatment Action Campaign.

[60] *Soobramoney v the Minister of Health, Kwazulu Natal,* 1998 (1) SA 776. (The Constitutional Court of South Africa held that the state was not constitutionally required to provide long-term renal dialysis treatment because the claimant fell outside the guidelines for medical eligibility and the exercise of the right to health, protected by Section 27 of the South African Constitution. Therefore the protection offered by section 27 can be reasonably limited by lack of resources.).

[61] *Williams v Jamaica,* Comm. No. 609/1995, U.N. Doc. CCPR/C/61/D/609/1995 (17 Nov 1997). (The Human Rights Committee held Jamaica responsible for denying a death row inmate adequate medical treatment for his mental condition as inhuman treatment contrary to Article 7, and as contrary to the respect for the inherent dignity of his person, protected by Article 10(1) of the International Covenant on Civil and Political Rights).

[62] *Jorge Odir Miranda Cortez et al v. El Salvador,* Case 12.249, Report No. 29/01, Inter-Am. C.H.R. OEA/Ser.L/V/II.111 Doc. 20 rev. at 284 (2000); *Juan Pablo et al. v Chile* (2001) Annual Report of the Inter-American Commission on Human Rights, OEO/Ser./L/V/II,114, doc 5 rev. 2001 (precautionary principle applied as an interim measure to require El Salvador and Chile respectively to provide treatment to those with HIV/AIDS pending decision on the merits of their claim to be entitled to treatment) (Inter-American Commission on Human Rights); *Eisler (Litigation Guardian of) v. Ontario* (2004) 234 D.L.R. (4th) 169 (application for an interlocutory injunction granted since the autistic children would suffer irreparable harm if their treatment were discontinued).

courts of law, or explain to judges how the outcomes of their policies protect the human rights of individuals.

However, courts in many countries have become more accessible to private initiatives to hold governments to legal account for health care policies and their consequences. Court have relaxed ancient legal doctrines, such as the offences of champerty and maintenance that prohibited third parties and special interest groups from maintaining or sponsoring private individuals to incur the financial costs of bringing litigation. Moreover, courts have become more accommodating of class action suits, and to allowing interventions in governmental proceedings by third parties appearing as friends of the court, called *amicus curiae*, to represent interests that the original parties to the litigation may fail to address or protect. Some jurisdictions, such as South Africa, have not left the justifiability of class actions to judicial benevolence, and have instead made specific provisions in their constitutions [63]. Many of these private initiatives were not only resisted by governmental administrations, but were also unfamiliar to the judges themselves, who were inclined to defer to governments on matters of resource allocation.

For instance, when private individuals or interest groups brought proceedings to require governmental funding of health care services, courts did not require governmental authorities even to explain the reasons on which their decisions were based. In a leading case in the English Court of Appeal, rejecting a parental claim for treatment of a 10-year old child with leukemia, it has been observed that:

> Difficult and agonizing judgments have to be made as to how a limited budget is best allocated to the maximum advantage of the maximum number of patients. That is not a judgment the court can make. In my judgment, it is not something that a health authority…can be fairly criticized for not advancing before the court [64].

This reasoning has been echoed by courts in other countries [65].

When courts were inclined to require or receive evidence of reasons, they were similarly disposed to observe that for them to mandate the supply of services from limited health care budgets would deny resources to other equally entitled individuals or interests that were not represented before the court. Judges recognize the polycentric nature of health systems, and understand that changing one part of the system will have ramifications in another part. It has been suggested that it might be 'improper for the court to make an order of mandamus compelling (a government authority) to do that…which it can do at the expense of others not before the court …'[66] The judges rules that a decision favorable to the initiators of such proceedings would risk causing injustice to the unrepresented interests. Accordingly, the court declined to entertain these claims on their merits.

Courts strictly applied the constitutional doctrine of Separation of Powers. As the English Court of Appeal has observed 'It is not for this court, or indeed any court, to substitute its own judgment for the judgment of those who are responsible for the allocation of

---

[63] South African Constitution, section 38©.

[64] *R v Cambridge Health Authority ex p. B,* [1995] 2 All E.R. 129, at 137 (Sir Thomas Bingham, M.R.).

[65] *Shortland v Northland Health* [1998] 1 NZLR 433 (CA) (The Court of Appeals of New Zealand upheld a lower court decision not to review a clinical determination to withhold long-term dialysis to a man with end stage renal failure because he was not a suitable candidate for dialysis.).

[66] *See R v Bristol Corporation,* ex Hendy [1974] 1 All E.R. 1047 at 1051 (Scarman LJ); for a commentary on this case, see Newdick 1996;119-135.

resources.'[67] The courts will intervene only in the event of 'a decision which is so outrageous of its defiance of logic or of accepted moral standards that no sensible person who had applied his mind to the question to be decided could have arrived at it' [68]. An additional argument is made that 'courts are not institutionally equipped to make the wide-ranging factual and political enquiries necessary...'[69] As a result, judges have tended to hold that the allocation of scarce public resources among competing interests must remain the responsibility of the executive branch of government, answerable only to the electorate, without general scrutiny by the judicial branch of government [70].

3.2. Scrutiny

Courts, however, are gradually moving from the practice of deference to government in matters of resource allocation, to a mode of scrutiny. Courts are recognizing that governments under the rule of law are bound to respect individual legal rights protected by national constitutions and international human rights treaties. Further, courts are now requiring greater transparency and rationality in governmental health policy making to ensure substantive and procedural fairness. As evidence-based medicine is emerging as the standard in clinical care, [71] so too is evidence-based health policy emerging as the standard for fairness in health systems. This will be increasingly the case as evidence-based decision-making (EBDM) continues to be applied in health care systems to promote best health care practices and effective delivery of health care [72]. It has been noted the 'EBDM has the potential-and far more potential than other decision-making methods-of creating a health care system that delivers not only excellent health care, but also great patient equality, autonomy and dignity. Accordingly, judicial review of health care decisions should use standards that promote EBDM'[73].

Canadian courts are moving in a direction of scrutiny, particularly as they apply the Canadian Charter of Rights and Freedoms in 1982, which gives domestic effect to the International Covenant on Civil and Political Rights. The Charter binds only government agencies. However, in *Eldridge v. British Columbia (Attorney General)*, the Supreme Court of Canada held that governments can not evade their Charter obligations by delegating responsibilities they have assumed to private agencies or corporation, such as public hospital, which despite substantial government funding, have legal status as private corporations [74]. Governments are legally bound to ensure that agencies discharging governmental functions, whether governmental agencies or private corporations, comply with individual rights and freedoms protected by the Charter. Accordingly, in *Eldridge,* the Supreme Court held the provincial government in breach of its Charter duties by permitting a hospital to discriminate against hearing impaired patients on grounds of their disability. The Court required the

---

[67] *R v. Secretary of State for Social Services,* ex p. Walker (1992), e B<LR 32, per Sir John Donaldson, MR at 35.
[68] Council of Civil Service Unions v. Minister for the Civil Service, [1985] AC 3 74, per Lord Diplock at 410.
[69] Treatment Action Campaign, par 27.
[70] *Syrett* 2004;289-321.
[71] Oxford Centre for Evidence-Based Medicine 2004.
[72] Dobrow et al 2004:207-217.
[73] Greschner 2005.
[74] *Stoffman v Vancouver General Hospital* [1990] 3 SCR 483 (Supreme Court of Canada).

government to submit a scheme for its approval that satisfies patients' right to care and treatment without discrimination.

The British Columbia Court of Appeal subsequently went further in *Auton (Guardian ad Litem of) v British Columbia (Attorney General)* holding the province's withholding of treatment for autistic children unconstitutionally discriminatory on grounds both of disability and age [75]. The Court found support in Canadian ratification of the Convention on the Rights of the Child [76], which is not incorporated into domestic law but which governments are judicially presumed to intend not to violate, because '[t]he Convention has moral force'[77]. The Court was not content to require the government to propose a scheme that would respect its legal responsibilities but mandated the government to fund a particular form of intensive behavioral therapy with a disputed success rate for particular pre-school age autistic children who fell outside the government's scheme of provision of services. This decision has been criticized as not requiring the plaintiff to produce sound scientific evidence of medical effectiveness of the disputed treatment. In so doing, the Court raised questions about what degree of effectiveness is required for a medical treatment to be publicly funded[78].

The Supreme Court of Canada is considering the government's appeal not only against the finding of Charter violation, but also against the Court of Appeal compelling funding of a particular form of intensive behavioral therapy with a disputed success rate. The government claimed it was answerable only to the electorate. This is a claim that the courts have traditionally accepted. However, it has been observed that:

> [w]hile in some circumstances excessive cost may justify a refusal to accommodate those with disabilities, one must be wary of putting too low a value on accommodating the disabled. It is all too easy to cite increased costs as a reason for refusing to accord the disabled equal treatment…Government agencies perform many expensive services for the public they serve [79].

The Supreme Court of Canada will accordingly have to decide in the *Auton* case if and how cost considerations justify overriding the executive branch's obligations under the Canadian Charter.

Governmental policies can be upheld by courts, not out of deference, but out of judges' independent assessments that they are justified, as the Constitutional Court of South Africa determined in the *Soobramoney* decision [80]. Where they are found not justified, however, courts can require that services be made fairly available, as the Constitutional Court ruled in the *Treatment Action Campaign* case [81]. That case concerned the public distribution of nevirapirine, a drug approved and registered by the Medicines Control Council of South Africa as safe and effective to reduce mother to child transmission of HIV. The case challenged the government policy that limited the public distribution of nevirapine to two

---

[75] *Auton (Guardian and Litem of) v British Columbia (Attorney General)* (2002) 220 D.L.R. (4th) 411 (B.C.C.A.) Ab appeal is pending before the Supreme Court of Canada.

[76] Convention on the Rights of the Child, 20 Nov 1989, GA Res. 44/25 (XLIV), UNGAOR, 44th Sess, Sipp. No. 49 at 167, UN Doc A/44/49, entered into force 1990; entered into force for Canada 12/01/92.

[77] Auton at 440.

[78] Greschner and Lewis 2003:501.

[79] *British Columbia (Superintendent of Motor Vehicles) v. British Columbia (Council of Human Rights)* [1993] 3 SCR 868 para 41 (Madam Justice (now Chief Justice) McLaughlin) (Supreme Court of Canada).

[80] Soobramoney v Minister of Health, KwaZulu-Natal, 1998 (1) SALR 765 (CC).

[81] Treatment Action Campaign.

public health facilities in each province. The claimants alleged that the government had acted unreasonably in

    a)   refusing to make nevirapine generally available to pregnant women with HIV in the public health sector for cases where it was thought to be medically indicated,

    b)   failing to establish a time frame for implementing a national program to prevent mother to child transmission of HIV [82].

The Constitutional Court of South Africa drew on their reasoning in *Grootbroom*, where they explained that national framework legislation on housing was insufficient because a coherent public program is necessary to ensure effective implementation of that legislation[83]. The Court reasoned that 'A Programme that excludes a significant segment of society cannot be said to be reasonable...'[84] In the *Treatment Action Campaign* decision, the Court applied this reasonableness standard to hold a Ministry of Health program that excluded 90% of pregnant women with HIV/AIDS from the public distribution of nevirapine unreasonable, and, therefore in violation of the constitutional right to health under Article 27[85].

In so doing, they rejected the minimum core approach of the Committee on Economic, Social and Cultural Rights, as first elaborated in their General Comment 3 [86]. The Court evidenced some uncertainty over what would constitute the particular elements of a minimum core of services in the circumstances of this case; '[I]t should be borne in mind that in dealing with such matters the Courts are not institutionally equipped to make the wide-ranging factual and political enquiries necessary for determining what the minimum-core standards...should be, nor for deciding how public revenues should be most effectively spent'[87]. The Court did not consider the further elaboration of the minimum core concept in General Comment 14 on the right to health in its judgment, even though it was adopted in 2000.

The Court explained the '...the socio-economic rights of the Constitution should not be construed as entitling everyone to demand that the minimum core be provided to them'[88]. Rather, the Court held that the obligation was to the progressive realization of rights: 'in its language, the Constitution accepts that it cannot solve all of our society's woes overnight....one of the limiting factors to the attainment of the constitution's guarantees is that of limited or scarce resources'[89]. The court explained that its 'function in respect of socio-economic rights is directed towards ensuring that legislative and other measures taken by the state are reasonable' [90]. The Court further elaborated:

> Courts are ill suited to adjudicate upon issues where Court orders could have multiple social and economic consequences for the community. The Constitution contemplates rather a restrained and focused role for the Courts, namely, to require the State to take measures to

---

[82] Treatment Action Campaign, par 2.

[83] *Republic of South Africa v Grootboom*, 2000 (11) BCLR 1169, pars 40-42 (The Constitutional Court of South Africa held that the national housing programme was in violation of the right to have access to adequate housing under Article 26 because it had no provision for those in desperate need.).

[84] Grootboom, par 43.

[85] Minister of Health v Treatment Action Campaign, par 80.

[86] Treatment Action Campaign, pars 26-39.

[87] Treatment Action Campaign, par 37.

[88] Treatment Action Campaign, par 34.

[89] Treatment Action Campaign, par 43.

[90] Treatment Action Campaign, par 36.

meet its constitutional obligations and to subject the reasonableness of these measures to evaluation. Such determination of reasonableness may in fact have budgetary implications, but are not in themselves directed at rearranging budgets. In this way the judicial, legislative and executive functions achieve appropriate constitutional balance [91].

However, they did not preclude the possibility of considering what others thought to be the minimum core for a particular economic, social and cultural rights in their determination of reasonableness under Article 27 of the South African Constitution [92].

The Courts in the *Treatment Action Campaign* decision missed the opportunity to consider the particular needs of pregnant women with HIV in its assessment of reasonableness of the program. The judges failed to explore whether neglecting the needs of pregnant women with HIV is discriminatory on grounds of sex, disability or possibly race under Article 9 on equality. Had the Court taken a more contextual approach to constitutional interpretation, it could have built upon its Article 9 jurisprudence on substantive equality, and in so doing apply the norms of the Women's Convention, which South Africa has ratified[93]. Their equality jurisprudence has specifically called for measures to address the continuing effects of past discriminatory wrongs:

> Particularly in a country such as South Africa, persons belonging to certain categories have suffered considerable unfair discrimination in the past. It is insufficient for the Constitution merely to ensure, through the Bill of Rights, that statutory provisions which have caused such unfair discrimination in the past are eliminated. Past unfair discrimination frequently has ongoing negative consequences, the continuation of which is not halted immediately when the initial causes thereof are eliminated, and unless remedied, may continue for a substantial time and even indefinitely...One could refer to such equality as remedial or restitutionary equality [94]

The General Recommendation on Women and Health which elaborates the content and meaning of Article 12 on health of the Women's Convention explains that neglecting to provide health care that only women need is a form of discrimination [95]. They might have also considered the intersections of different grounds of discrimination, including sex, health status and possibly race. The opportunity was also missed to build on the General Recommendation on Gender-related dimensions of racial discrimination [96] made by the Committee on the Elimination of Racial Discrimination, under the International Convention on the Elimination of All Forms of Racial Discrimination, which South Africa has ratified[97].

In acknowledging the particular form and manifestation of discrimination against women marginalized by sex, race and health status in accessing nevirapine, the Court would have at least placed government health officials on notice that such manifestations warrant careful scrutiny. Had the Court addressed the barriers that women face in accessing health care in the

---

[91] Treatment Action Campaign, par 38.

[92] Treatment Action Campaign, par 34.

[93] Ratification date for South Africa to the Women's Convention, 14/01/96.

[94] National Coalition for Gay and Lesbian Equality v Minister of Justice 1999 (1) SA 6 (CC) AT 38-39 per Ackerman J.

[95] CEDAW General Recommendation 24.

[96] Committee on the Elimination of Racial Discrimination, General Recommendation 25, AUGAOR 2000, UN Doc. A/55/18, Annex V, 152.

[97] South African ratification of the Convention on the Elimination of All Forms of Racial Discrimination, 9/01/99.

way they addressed the 'most urgent' needs of children in accessing nevirapine [98], they could have signaled that governments have obligations to accommodate women's particular needs. It is through the acknowledgment of its different forms and manifestations that discrimination can be recognized, identified and effectively addressed.

The Women's Health Report 1998 concludes that 'Women's health is inextricably linked to their status in society. It benefits from equality and suffers from discrimination'[99]. Had the Constitutional Court been inspired to acknowledge the discriminatory dimensions of the governments program, it would have moved well beyond the jurisprudence developed by courts in other countries on the constraints faced by women and girls in accessing health care. Courts have helpfully eliminated requirements for partners' authorization for provision of care to women [100], and parental consent requirements regarding mature adolescent girls [101]. Rulings have generally held that such third party authorization requirements violate the right to private life.

These decisions prohibiting third party authorization requirements are based on liberal theories of justice that tend to address only what governments must not do. The courts might have considered what positive provisions are needed to ensure that women can actually exercise their autonomy in ways that will protect and promote their health. Courts might come to consider how the patriarchal nature of authorization requirements produced women's vulnerability to ill health and disadvantage within the health care system [102]. It would have been a significant contribution to jurisprudence had courts examined how such requirements reproduce patriarchy, and what governments should do to change patriarchal values that obstruct women's access to health care.

Advocates and legal scholars face the challenge to guide courts to go beyond liberal theories of autonomy, in order to consider positive measures that can be taken to acknowledge the discriminatory harms that persist in the realities of women's lives. Progress might be achieved, for instance, if governments were required to train health officials to examine, through human rights needs assessments and gender analysis, how women's health needs can be accommodated in fact.

Courts in some countries have declined to require public health ministries to make emergency contraception available [103], while in others litigation is pending [104]. In still others,

---

[98] Treatment Action Campaign, pars 74-79, Sections 28(1)(b) and (c) on children's rights to access to basic health care.

[99] World Health Organization 1998:8.

[100] A v B, 35 (iii) P.D. 57 (Supreme Court of Israel, 1981): *Attorney-General (QLD) ex rel. Kerr* v T, 46 ALR 275 (High Court of Australia, 1983): C. V S., 2 W.L.R. 1108 (Court of Appeal, England, 1987): *Judgement* of Feb. 15, 1978, Dec. No. 157/77, 3 Yugoslz Law 65 (Constitutional Court of Yugoslavia, 1979); *Judgement* of Oct. 31, 1980, Conseil d'Etat, D.S. Jus. 19,732 (Council of State of France, 1980); *Judgement* of Mar 31, 1988, Corte Cost., Gass. Ufficiale, 1 serie speciale, April 13, 1988, n.15; Giur. Cost. E Civ. 2110 (Constitutional Court of Italy, 1988); *Kelly v Kelly*, 2 FLR 828 (Court of Session, Scotland) (1997); *Planned Parenthood v Danforth*, 428 U.S. 52, 69 (Supreme Court of the United States, 1976; *Tremblay v Daigle*, 62 D.L.R. (4th) 634, 665 (Supreme Court of Canada, 1989).

[101] Gillick v West Norfolk and Wisbech Area Health Authority [1986] AC 112 (House of Lords).

[102] Standing 1997:2.

[103] Sara Phillipi et al. v Ministerio de Salud, Instituto de Salud Publica and Laboratorio Silesia (2001), Supreme Court 2186-2001, August 30th, 2001 (supreme Court of Chile).

[104] *Ages v Instituto de Salud Publica* (2004) 20°Juzgado Civil, rol 5839-02; Ages v Instuto de Salud Publica, (2004) Santiago Court of Appeals, rol 4200-03 (an appeal against a lower court decision to ban an emergency contraceptive product and a stay of that opinion is pending before the Santiagl Court of Appeals of Chile; *Carlos Humberto Gomez Arambula* (File No 88119) (a declaration is sought to invalidate the Resolution 266285 approving the emergency contraception, Postinor 2, by Ministry of Social Security's National Institute

however, courts have explained that failure adequately to disclose an emergency contraceptive option within 72 hours of women's unprotected intercourse, when competent practitioners would have provided information about that option, will justify awards of damages for negligence if women show that they would have taken the option, and that they have suffered injury as a consequence of the option being denied [105].

Legal application of a tort or delictual standard of care to provision of emergency contraception is an important step to ensure that women have the necessary information to make informed choices about their care. As against this application, courts have often failed even to consider the impact on maternal mortality and morbidity of prohibition on emergency contraception, and the manifold harms women face from violation of their rights to liberty and security of the person, and to non-discrimination. Judges have ignored scientific facts that show that emergency contraception can act only to prevent pregnancy, simply stating that emergency contraception is a form of abortion. Scientific evidence shows, however, that it prevents pregnancy, and is of no effect after pregnancy has occurred [106].

Denial takes many forms [107]. Denial of women's human rights to medically indicated health services is marked by misrepresentation of scientific facts, by refusal to recognize the history of women's oppression and denying responsibility for past and present practices that violate women's rights. Courts have a significant role to play in overcoming these many forms of denial by:

- acknowledging health-related violations, whether it be against women or, for example, those marginalized by race and ethnicity [108],
- requiring public accountability for those violations, and
- formulating appropriate measures to remedy such violations [109].

---

of Vigilance for Medicines and Food (INVIMA) (Council of State of Colombia, Administrative Law Seciont); *Juan Carlos Barrera* (File No. 17.806) (appeal might be sought against the decision of Sept 30, 2004 that an action of Protection (Tutela) in the name of the non-born (nasciturus) against Profamilia for distributing emergency contraception with Levonorgestrel 0.75mg and the pharmaceutical laboratories that produce medicines using the Levonorgestrel 0.75mg and the pharmaceutical laboratories that produce medicines using the Levonorgestrel 0.75 mg as an active principle (Schering, Wyeth, HRA Pharma, Leiras; Gedeon Richter) is the proper mechanism to challenge the approval of INVIMA of emergency contraception with Levonorgestrel 0.75 mg is not the proper means to impugn the proceedings of a general character (Colombian Supreme Court of Justice-Penal Chamber).

[105] *Kathleen Brownfield v Daniel Freeman Marina Hospital* (1989) 208 Cal. App 3d 405, 412, 413 (California Court of Appeals, 2nd Appellate District (div 4) explained that failure to adequately disclose an emergency contraceptive option within 72hours of unprotected intercourse, when a skilled practitioner would have provided information about the option, can justify an award an award of damages for negligence if the woman shows that she would have taken that option, and suffered injury as a consequence of the option not being offered).

[106] Grimes and Raymond 2002:181.

[107] International Council on Human Rights Policy 2000.

[108] Randall 1995:147-224; Chapman and Rubenstein (eds) 1998.

[109] Boven 200:111-133.

4. THE USE OF TEMPORARY SPECIAL MEASURES TO PROMOTE EQUALITY IN HEALTH

Given the disparities in health status, whether measured by structural, process or outcome indicators [110], among different subgroups of population, it might be necessary for ministries of health and courts to consider the use of affirmative action measures to promote fairness and substantive equality in health care reform. Generally speaking, affirmative action is based on temporary positive measures intended to increase opportunities for health advancement for historically and systemically disadvantaged groups. The Women's Convention described affirmative action as temporary special measures, and explains in Article 4(1) that:

Adoption...of temporary special measures aimed at accelerating de facto equality between men and women shall not be considered discrimination..., but shall in no way entail as a consequence the maintenance of unequal or separate standards; these measures shall be discontinued when the objectives of equality of opportunity and treatment have been achieved.

Article 4(1) is explanatory in nature. It distinguishes permissible temporary special measures, aimed at achieving *de facto* or substantive equality, from otherwise discriminatory measures [111]. It explains that, if States do take such measures, they will not be considered discriminatory [112], provided that the measures satisfy the following three tests:

First, they must accelerate equality in fact,

Second, they must not entail the maintenance of unequal or separate standards, and

Third, they must be discontinued when the objectives of equality of opportunity and treatment have been achieved [113].

Temporary special measures can range from small initiatives that encounter little resistance, such as provision of health promotion information, to more costly training programs, and, finally, to more controversial measures, such as programs to facilitate access of high risk groups to necessary health services until such time as those groups are at no more that the ordinary risk in the general population. The more targeted and robust the measures are, the more contested they become.

According to Article 12(1) of the Women's Convention, courts may find that temporary special measures are required where such measures are the most 'appropriate...to eliminate discrimination against women in the field of health care...' The criteria for determining which measures are 'appropriate' to eliminate discrimination against women are more difficult to determine in the field of health than in such areas as participation in political and public life, and access to education and employment, where affirmative action measures have been frequently used.

The success of affirmative action is often measured by the degree to which men and women are recruited equally into the work force and educational institutions, because

---

[110] Interim Report of Special Rapporteur 2003.

[111] Committee on the Elimination of Discrimination against Women (CEDAW), General Recommendation No.25, on article 4(1) of the Convention on the Elimination of All Forms of Discrimination against Women, on termporary Special Measures, CEDAW/C/2004/I/WP.1/Rev.1, 30Jan2004 CEDAW, par 18.

[112] This view is also taken by the Human Rights Committee in its General Comment 18: Non-discrimination at par 10 HRI/Gen/1/Rev.4 (2000).

eligibility for employment and education does not usually depend on differences in sex. However, in matters of health, the issue is not only one of treating equal eligibility equally, but also of reacting appropriately to biological and physiological differences between the sexes and the underlying social conditions that affect the sexes differently. That is, temporary special measures are generally used to ensure that similar cases are treated in similar ways. Such measures have not commonly been used to ensure that different situations or conditions are treated fairly according to those differences. As a result, temporary special measures might be more usefully applied to require equality in access to specific therapeutic drugs and services among subgroups of women, as measured by process indicators.

A focus of the Women's Convention is on the elimination of all forms of discrimination against women, including multiple forms. Where subgroups of women are differentiated by health indicators, especially process and outcome indicators, and those health indicators correlate, for instance, with race, ministries of health might use temporary special measures. Such measures might well be appropriate to address discrimination on the compounded grounds of race and sex, where such measures are proportional to the end of achieving substantive equality in access to specified treatment among subgroups.

It is unlikely that courts will order temporary special measures to address the underling socio-economic conditions because the evidence of the effectiveness of addressing such conditions is more complex, indeterminate and variable. In this sense, the law in general and temporary special measures in particular are limited in achieving substantive equality in the health context because of their inability to address the underlying socio-economic conditions[114]

5. CONCLUSION

As courts move from a mode of deference to governmental authority to a mode of deliberation on governmental responsibility enforceable by law, they will play an increasingly important role in generating thoughtful and informed debate about fairness in health care reform. Health care decisions can no longer be protected by governmental political choices or concealed behind veils of clinical or scientific judgments or cost-effective assessments. Health care reform has to be planned and undertaken in a transparent manner, and needs to comply with principles of fairness embodied in constitutions and human rights treaties.

Greater dialogue is needed among all sectors of society about fairness in health care reform. Where judicial review is understood as a dialogue among judges, governments and legislatures [115], evidenced-based health assessments are necessary to inform the debate. Health professionals have to engage with wider audiences concerned with equity and human right issues more generally. Moreover, courts have to ensure that their decisions are grounded in sound understandings of clinical care, health systems and underlying determinants of health, and have to provide objective reasons why particular reforms will achieve greater fairness. Courts will always be sensitive to their particular institutional role and capacities

---

[113] General Recommendation 25, pars 18-24.
[114] Ngwena 2000:111-131,126.
[115] Fitzpatrick Slye 2003:669-680,680; Roach 2004.

relative to other branches of government, and will continue to carve out a 'restrained and focused role'[116] in resource allocation decisions.

Health care reform cannot be debated in a normative vacuum. Reforms need to be evidenced-based, and grounded in principles of fairness ad justice. Where reforms are not evidenced-based, publicly understood or justified, they may be challenged through the courts by the application of constitutional and human rights values.

REFERENCES

Beauchamp,TL; Childress, FL. *Principles of biomedical ethics 5th ed*, Oxford: Oxford University Press; 2001.

Braveman, P. Monitoring equity in health and healthcare: a conceptual framework. *J Health Popul Nutr*, 2003 21, 181-192.

Braveman, P; Gruskin, S. Poverty, equity, human rights and health. *Bulletin of WHO*, 2003a 81, 583.

Braveman, P; Gruskin, S. Defining equity in health. *J Epidemiol Community Health*, 2003b 57,254-258.

Chapman, AR. Core obligations related to the right to health. In: Chapman, A; Russell, S editors. *Core obligations: Building a framework for economic, social and cultural rights.* Antwerp: Intersentia; 2002; 185-215.

Chapman, AR; Rubinstein, LS. *Human rights and health: The legacy of apartheid.* Washington, DC: Association for the Advancement of Science; 1998.

Commission on the Future of Health Care in Canada. *Building on values: The future of health care in Canada – Final Report* Saskatoon: Commission on the Future of Health Care in Canada; 2002.

Commission on Human Rights. *Note by the Secretary General: Interim Report of the Special Rapporteur of the Commission on Human Rights on the Right of Everyone to the Enjoyment of the Highest Attainable Standard of Physical and Mental Health*, Mr. Paul Hunt A/58/427, 10 Oct 2003.

Cook, RJ; Dickens, BM; Fathalla, MF. *Reproductive health and human rights: integrating medicine, ethics and law.* Oxford: Clarendon; 2003.

Dahlgren, G; Whitehead, M. *Policies and strategies to promote equity in health.* Copenhagen: WHO Regional Office; 1991.

Daniels, N. Benchmarks of fairness for health care reform: a policy tool for developing countries. Bulletin of WHO, 2000a 78(6),740-750, online: *http://www.who.int/docstore/ bulletin/pdf/2000/issue6/0583.pdf* (accessed: 11May2004.

Daniels, N; Kennedy, B; Kawachi, I. *Is inequality bad for our health?* Boston: Beacon Press; 2000b.

Daniels, N; Light, DW; Caplan, RL. *Benchmarks of fairness for health care reform.* New York: Oxford University Press; 1996.

Dobrow, M; Goel, V; Reg, U. Evidence-based health policy: Context and utilization. *Social Science and Medicine*, 2004 58, 207-217.

---

[116] Treatment Action Campaign at par 38.

Doyal, L. Gender equity in health: debates and dilemmas. *Social Science and Medicine*. 2000 51, 931-939.

Fitzpatrick, J; Slye, RC. Economic and social rights-South Africa – Role of international standards in interpreting and implementing constitutionally guaranteed rights. *American Journal of International law*, 2003 97, 669-680.

Flood, CM. *International health care reform: a legal, economic, and political analysis*. London: Routledge; 2000.

Ford, CA; Millstein, SG; Halpern-Felsher, BL; Irwin, CE. Influence of physician confidentiality assurances on adolescents' willingness to disclose information and seek future health care. *Journal of the American Medical Association*, 1997 278, 1029-1034.

Gomez-Jauregui, J; Daniels, N; Reichenbach, L. Cervical cancer screening program in Mexico: Equity and fairness implications. *Working Paper, Center for Population and Development Studies*, Harvard School of Public Health. 2004.

Gostin, LO; Lazzarini, Z. *Human rights and public health in the AIDS pandemic*. New York: Oxford; 1997.

Greschner, D. Charter rights and evidence-based decision-making in the health care system: Toward a symbiotic relationship. In: Flood editor. *Just Medicare: What's In, What's Out, Who Decides*, Toronto: University of Toronto Press; 2006.

Greschner, D; Lewis, S. Auton and evidence-based decision-making. *Canadian Bar Review. Medicare in the Courts*. 2003 82, 501-

Grimes, DA; Raymond, EG. Emergency contraception. *Ann Intern Med*, 2002 137, 180-189.

Health Canada. Certain circumstances: issues in equity and responsiveness in access to health care in Canada (Ottawa: Health Canada, 2001), online: *http://www.hc-sc.gc.ca/hppb/healthcare/pdf/circumstances.pdf* (accessed: 11May2004).

Health Canada. Exploring concepts of gender and health. Ottawa: Health Canada. Online: *http://www.hc.sc.gc.ca/english/women/pdf/exploring_concepts.pdf* (accessed: 12 May 2004). Health Policy and Planning, 2003 12, 1-18.

International Council on Human Rights Policy. The persistence and mutation of racism. Versoix, Switzerland; 2004. at 6-8, online at *www.ichrp.org* (accessed 20September2004).

Lacey, N. Feminist legal theory and the rights of Women. In: Knop, K editor. *Gender and human rights*. Oxford: Oxford University Press; 2003, 13-55.

Newdick, C. *Who should we treat?* Oxford: Clarendon Press; 1996.

Ngwena, C. Substantive equality in South African health care: the limits of the law. *Medical Law International*, 2000 4, 111-131.

Oxford Centre for Evidence-Based Medicine. Levels of evidence and grades of recommendation. 2004. *www.cebm.net/levels_of_evidence.asp* (Accessed 3October2004).

Raday, F. Systematizing the application of different types of temporary special measures under article 4 of CEDAW. In: Boerefijn, F; Coomans, J; Holtmaat, GR; Wolleswinkiel, R editors. *Temporary special measures – Accelerating de facto equality of women under Article 4(1) CEDAW*. Antwerp: Intersentia Publishers; 2003; 35-44.

Randall, VR. Racist health care: reforming an unjust health care system to meet the needs of African-Americans. In: Grubb, A; Mehlman, MJ editors. *Justice and health care: Comparative perspectives*. Chichester: John Wiley; 1995; 147-224.

Roach, K. *Constitutional, remedial and international dialogues about rights: the Canadian experience*. Faculty of Law, University of Toronto; 2004. Unpublished workshop paper.

Standing, H. Gender and Equity in health sector reform programmes: a review. *Health Policy Plan,* 1997 12, 1-18.

Syrett, K. Deference or deliberation: rethinking the judicial role in the allocation of healthcare resources. Proceedings of the 15th World Congress on Medical law, Congress Proceedings. Sydney Australia, 2004, 190-198.

Syrett, K. Impotence or importance? Judicial review in an era of explicit NHS rationing. *Modern Law Review,* 2004 67(2), 289-321.

Tuohy, CH. *Accidental logics: the dynamics of change in the health care arena in the United States. Britain and Canada*: Oxford University Press; 1999.

Van Boven, T. Discrimination and human rights law: Combating racism. In: Redman, S editor. *Discrimination and human rights: the case of racism.* Oxford: Oxford University Press; 2001; 111-133.

Van Rensburg, HCJ. *Health and health care in South Africa.* Pretoria: Van Schaik; 2004.

World Health Organization. World health report 1998. *Life in the 21st Century: A vision for all.* Geneva: WHO; 1998.

In: Women's Health in the Majority World: Issues and Initiatives   ISBN1-1-60021-493-2
Eds: L. Elit and J. Chamberlain Froese, pp. 133-137   © 2007 Nova Science Publishers, Inc.

Chapter 7

THE ROLE OF EDUCATION ON WOMEN'S HEALTH AND WOMEN'S RIGHTS

Sima Samar[1]

Afghanistan Independent Human Rights Commission

ABSTRACT

Background

The women of Afghanistan faced one of the worst situations in terms of their near enslavement and violation of rights. The importance of education to reverse this trend will be reviewed.

Methods

Eight reasons for the oppression of women such as lack of access to justice and misrepresentation of religion will be reviewed. Nine areas for development such as education and access to reproductive health care will be discussed.

Discussion

For Afghan women to enter the 21st century as productive and healthy members of society, education will play a pivotal role.

INTRODUCTION

As it is well publicized by now, the women of Afghanistan face one of the worst situations in terms of their near enslavement and violation of rights. Unfortunately, this situation is not unique. I will relate the experience of Afghan women in the context of

---
[1] Corresponding author's Email: sima_samar@yahoo.com

highlighting the crisis and problems that are endemic to their own particular situation but can be extended to all women in the region. Based on these, I will offer a broad outline for strategies that will help to implement the gender mainstreaming and Millennium Development Goal's (MDG) in Afghanistan. These include: gender equality, role of education in every aspect of the life and especially in health. . ˙

Afghanistan has always been a patriarchal society, but in the '60s and '70s women began to make some progress. However, three decades of war destroyed most of these advances. Fundamentalism was built and supported by outside countries as the strategy to fight the Soviet Invasion. This strategy had horrible consequences for women. These are consequences we live with every day as we try to rebuild our country and women's lives.

Widespread illiteracy and lack of education was one of the main reasons why the war in Afghanistan has been so violent and lasted so long. Education is as basic human right. Education is necessary in order to bring the culture of war to an end and to achieve sustainable peace. Education is necessary for the reconstruction of Afghanistan. Indeed, education is necessary if we want to talk about creating a healthy society. If we do not have healthy mothers, the children will not be healthy, the society will not be healthy, and finally the world will not be healthy. Also, with out education, we cannot talk about gender mainstreaming and achieving the millennium development goals. If education is just a word on paper, it will not help to improve the lives of women.

The women's rights situation in Afghanistan is somewhat better today than during the wars. Women are now able to work and girls can attend school. The demand for girls and women's education is greater than ever. The illiteracy rate in our country is 85% for women.

Besides the widespread lack of education, the reasons for the oppression of women in our country and also in the broader region can be isolated as:

a) Lack of Education and lack of awareness about their rights and about their own status: Even if they have the rights to education and the equal rights in the constitution, they may not be aware of their entitlement lack of awareness always reason to the subordination of women and girls in Afghanistan.

b) Although girls are going to schools since the fall of Taliban government, the number of girls that attend are less then the half of the numbers of the boys.

c) The Misuse of Religion and culture in our society: As the women do not know much about their status in Islam, the men always try to misuse Islam and culture to be able to control the women in the society. Men have their own beliefs and this is painted with an Islamic value, though the practices may have no roots in Islam at all. For example, the culture of *Bad,* is the attempt to solve the problem between the families by victimizing girls in order to solve these disputes. *Bad* is clearly against the Islamic values, because in Islam the women have to consent to marry any person and it is indeed an important part of the marriage. In the practice of *Bad*, the girls are almost never consented, neither are they entitled to know the individual to whom they are getting married to. Hence, to all intents and purposes, she is traded as a slave by her own family and treated as such by her in-laws. What will ultimately happen is that she will not be a healthy person and she will not be able to bring up healthy children. It will be very difficult to trade an educated girl in this way.

d) Lack of Access to Justice: Afghanistan is a very patriarchal society; there is a high likelihood that the judge or prosecutor will be uneducated and bear little sensitivity or sympathy to the issues of women's rights. In most of the cases, a woman may not even be able to reach the court. Even if she does gain access, she will not be treated well and may be further victimized and harassed because the definition of a good woman in our country corresponds to a woman who bears all her problems and she never protests. If she protests or goes to court and demands justice she is treated as a bad woman. An educated women cares about the definition of bad women, but she would also value and seek out justice.

e) Lack of Accesses to Reproductive Health Care: The ongoing war has destroyed much of the health system in the country that was not much to begin with. As a result, the majority of women do not have access to reproductive health care. They usually end up bearing at least 8-10 children. A mother in this circumstance is often very weak and naturally preoccupied with her own health or that of her children. Therefore, she cannot think about all the other problems and take part in issues outside of the home.

f) Poverty: Poverty is a problem of oppression of women and weak health. The status of a woman is degraded because her parents sell her; when she goes to the husband's family, she is treated as a property and she is made to work as a slave to survive. In such a situation, a woman has little chance to even nominally educate herself. Her economical dependency causes her to be second-class person in home and the society.

g) Women's Limitation in Political Decision Making or at Policy Making Level: Afghanistan has always been a male dominated society and men are responsible for making all the decisions so it is very natural that women's issues are ignored. Even in cases where nominal attempts are made at improving the lot of women, they do not take women's problem seriously and the policies may not necessarily favor women.

h) Lack of Women's Participation in Peace Process: The situation that developed during and after the war in Afghanistan has very much reflected a male dominated culture. When the Bonn agreement was being formulated and the future of Afghanistan was being laid out, there were no women as active participants in the process. Although women made up 42% of the vote for the presidential and parliamentary election, there are only 26% women representative in parliament. The majority of Afghan women do not enjoy basic human rights and their daily life has not changed much.

i) Lack of Security: The main problem for women in our country is lack of security. During the 25 years of war and conflict, women are the first group that were and are victimized. Since men were holding the gun, they had more power to control the women's movement. Even now where we have so called peace in Afghanistan, women have absolutely no say in the security of their country. Security is more of a problem for women than men. In every country in conflict, women are used as toll to win the war.

If we really want to empower the women and implement gender equality, or more ambitiously, make some headway in solving the problems facing this world, we cannot ignore that half of the population in every sector of society are women. Education has a clear role in solving the problems.

These issues have to be given serious consideration, and I recommend the following for Afghanistan as part of the global human body.

1. Education is the key for healthy society. Education will allow women full participation in their development: Education should be provided at all levels in Afghanistan. As we all know, the female population was denied their basic human rights of access to education. The war factions paid little attention to education in the country during the 23 years of war. So education for girls of all ages is required. In order to change the mentality of the society, we have to educate the men and provide educational facilities to boys so that they may have a valuable alternative to the *madrasas* (religious schools). While the media shows that millions of Afghan girls are going to school, they fail to show the actual percentage of girls who have access to education and the quality of the facilities and teaching at these schools.

2. Security: As I mentioned before, security is one of the biggest problem in our country. Since December 2001 when I went back to Afghanistan, we have been consistently asking for more ISAF troops in our country. The international community has to support Afghanistan, but unfortunately the security situation in Afghanistan is getting worse in the last year. As a result, in some part of the country only 3% of the children who are going to schools are girls. In the past year, almost 300 schools were burnt or closed. Most of these were girls' schools. The fundamentalist understand that if the Afghan girls are educated, they will not be able to control them.

3. Education in Islamic Principles and Islamic Values: Extensive education in Islamic principles and values must be provided to the sources of religious guidance. This will be an important step in avoiding the misuse of Islam, which is a very peaceful religion. With proper education, these religious authorities can become an important ally in battling violence against women and support to implement the human rights and women rights conventions and treaty in the country. In fact, Islam started with word *Iqra* which means read. In Islam, education is compulsory for every Muslim woman and man.

4. Access to Health Care: Access to health care must be considered a basic human right, especially reproductive health care for women. In order to encourage women to actively participate in the reconstruction of Afghanistan, she cannot also try to care for 10 children. Without the health of women in a country assured, we cannot have a healthy nation. It is very clear that the educated women do understand their health problems and they are able to control the number of their children. The educated women understand about their bodies and they can make informed decision about their reproductive choices. This will be a crucial part in reducing poverty.

5. Participation in the Peace Process and Decision Making: Women's participation in the peace processes and decision-making is very important, and their role should not be a mere symbolic role. Their role should be critical and active. Women cannot play a participatory role in the peace process if they do not have an education. Affirmative action and positive discrimination is needed.

6. Equal Rights and Guarantees: It is very important to have equal rights in the constitution and the national laws. Still crucial is to make these laws and regulations

a reality for the women in any country. The solubility of these laws must also be accompanied by the deployment of sensitive and trained female and male judges and lawyers to implement the law. To make all these steps a reality in Afghanistan, we need and insist on good quality education. All the governments must be pushed to ratify and abide the international standards of human rights and be accountable for them.

7. Economic Empowerment: Economic empowerment of women is another crucial issue in giving women a chance to participate in society. In order to give economic opportunity to the women, education plays an important role.

8. The other very important issue in Afghanistan is to protect human rights and women's' rights by pushing for effective law enforcement: At the moment, guns still rule the country and a culture of impunity is prevalent. To this end, the international community has to help Afghanistan in law enforcement. International participation in law enforcement in Afghanistan will be crucial if the international community wants to achieve a sustainable peace in Afghanistan and curtail the problems in Afghanistan from spreading beyond our boundaries. Women's participation on law making is important and the law should not be discriminatory to the women.

9. Finally access to good quality education is basic human right. Every person has the right to receive an education. Without an education, it is impossible to build the health system and provide health services to the people in any country. Education is the only way to change the mentality in the society. Lack of education will create an environment for fundamentalism, terrorism and all kind of crimes.

Access to health care is also basic human rights. For women access to reproductive health is vital to be able to bring healthy child and secure the feature of this world and the human dignity. Health and education has very close links and connection to each other, in fact they compensate each other.

Development is not possible with out education and peace. Peace and development will not be possible with out women's active participation. Women will not be safe with out access to reproductive health care and access to contraception.

Finally with out education the Human security, and human rights will not be granted. We need security, social justice and non-violent world for our feature generation.

In: Women's Health in the Majority World: Issues and Initiatives   ISBN1-1-60021-493-2
Eds: L. Elit and J. Chamberlain Froese, pp. 139-154   © 2007 Nova Science Publishers, Inc.

Chapter 8

PARTNERING FOR REPRODUCTIVE HEALTH: SOGC'S INTERNATIONAL EXPERIENCE

*A. B. Lalonde[1] and L. Perron[2],**

[1]Dept Obs/Gyn, University of Ottawa,
Society of Obstetricians and Gynaecology of Canada (SOGC), Canada
FIGO Safe Motherhood and Newborn Health Committee
[2]International Women's Health Program, SOGC, Canada

ABSTRACT

Health professionals, including obstetricians and gynaecologists, have a strong tradition of involvement in international women's health initiatives in lower resurce countries. These contributions, often initiated by individual professionals through formal but often-informal collaborations, are the basis of the involvement of the Society of Obstetricians and Gynaecologists of Canada (SOGC) in international women's health.

In 1998, the Society committed to pursue excellence in international women's health and to focus its efforts on promoting universal access to emergency obstetric care, as a means to reduce maternal and newborn mortality and morbidity worldwide. Its areas of expertise include increasing access and quality of maternal and newborn health services, including safer pregnancy and delivery and building capacity of professional associations to assume leadership in the field. Its activities are supported by the professional expertise of its members who volunteer as trainers and technical consultants.

This chapter will provide an overview of the international program of the SOGC. It will explore: (a) the contribution of professional associations in global and national efforts to reduce maternal and newborn mortality and morbidity; (b) the partnership model of the Society and its experience in enhancing capacity of professional associations from lower resource countries to assume leadership in the field of sexual and reproductive health; (c) the value of partnerships between professional associations from higher and lower resource countries for the purpose of building capacity.

---

*Contact: Liette Perron, SOGC, 780, promenade Echo Drive, Ottawa, ON K1S 5R7, Canada, Phone: (613) 730-4192 ext 223, Fax: 613 730-4314, Email: *lperron@sogc.com*.

INTRODUCTION

"For us, obstetricians and midwives [...] maternal mortality is not statistics. It is not numbers.... Maternal mortality is [...] women, women who have names, women who have faces, and we have seen these faces in the throes of agony, distress and despair. They are faces that continue to live in your memory and to haunt your dreams. And this is not simply because these are young women who die in the prime of their lives [...] And it is not simply because a maternal death is one of the most terrible ways to die, be it bleeding to death, the convulsions of toxaemia of pregnancy, the unbearable pangs of obstructed labour or the agony of puerperal sepsis [...] It is not for all of this that maternal mortality is such a human tragedy. It is because in almost each and every case, in retrospect, it is an event that could have been prevented. It is an event that should never have been allowed to happen. It is an event that bears and should bear so heavily on our collective conscience."

Mahmoud Fatthala, FIGO [1]

In the last decade, professional associations concerned with women's health have joined the global movement calling for the reduction of maternal and neonatal mortality and morbidity. Although international professional associations have been most visible in this area, their national affiliates are increasingly involved as leaders and viewed as important stakeholders in national efforts to promote safer pregnancy and childbirth.

The Society of Obstetricians and Gynaecologists of Canada (SOGC) is a voluntary, non-profit professional organization dedicated to the promotion of optimal women's health through leadership, collaboration, education, research and advocacy in the practice of obstetrics and gynaecology in Canada. As a leading Canadian authority on reproductive health issues, the SOGC establishes national practice guidelines and provides medical education to more than 3,000 Canadian obstetricians/gynaecologists and other health professionals including family physicians, midwives and nurses. It is also increasingly involved in public education and awareness initiatives aimed at educating the Canadian public on a variety of domestic and international issues related to sexual and reproductive health. Since 1998, SOGC has supported professional associations in lower resource countries to strengthen their capacity to promote maternal and newborn health.

The Society is currently involved in a partnership initiative with the *Asociation de Gynecologia y Obstetricia de Guatemala* (AGOG), *la Société Haïtienne d'Obstétrique et Gynécologie* (SHOG) and the Association of Obstetricians and Gynaecologists of Uganda (AOGU). Funded by the Canadian International Development Agency (CIDA), the partnership program has supported the professional associations in developing leadership in initiatives aimed at reducing maternal and neonatal mortality and morbidity in their countries.

INCREASING ACCESS TO SKILLED CARE AT DELIVERY

Despite today's knowledge and technology, more than 529,000 women continue to die each year due to complications of pregnancy or childbirth. Furthermore, 3.3 million babies are stillborn, and more than four million others die within 28 days of birth. More than 99% of the maternal deaths and most of the neonatal deaths occur in lower income countries where access to maternal and newborn care is not available. Although globally 61.1% of births are attended by skilled professionals, in sub-Saharan Africa, barely 40% of women give birth assisted by skilled attendants. Also, nearly three quarters of all neonatal deaths could be prevented if women were adequately nourished and accessed appropriate care during pregnancy, childbirth and the postnatal period [2].

Since the 1987 Nairobi Safe Motherhood Conference, health professionals involved in obstetrics, and by extension their professional associations, have assumed leadership in promoting universal access to safe motherhood and newborn health. This commitment, reaffirmed at the 1997 Sri Lanka Conference, coincided with increasing evidence that most maternal and newborn deaths occur because women deliver their babies on their own or without skilled attendance and lack access to emergency obstetric care when faced with complications. Women also die due to complications related to unsafe abortions. Skilled care at birth, including emergency obstetric care, is a key intervention promoted globally to reduce the high rates of maternal and neonatal mortality which persist in many parts of the world. This policy shift toward ensuring the presence of skilled attendance at birth was further supported by the recognition that the international efforts to ensure training of traditional birth attendants had made little or no impact by itself on the reduction of maternal mortality and morbidity globally [3].

ROLE OF PROFESSIONAL ASSOCIATIONS

The International Federation of Gynaecology and Obstetrics (FIGO) and the International Confederation of Midwives (ICM) actively participated in the development and promotion of the strategy related to skilled attendance at birth and advocated for the participation of their national affiliates in the global movement for making pregnancy and childbirth safer. In a joint statement with the World Health Organization (WHO), they called for health professionals involved in maternal and newborn health to work collaboratively in ensuring quality of care and urged professional associations to assume "the responsibility to advocate for and [...] ensure [...] equitable access to high-quality care for all pregnant women and newborns in all circumstances and situations, irrespective of whether the care is being provided via private for-profit, private not-for-profit, or public services" [4].

Obstetricians/gynaecologists and midwives are strategically well placed to promote maternal and newborn health and work toward the reduction of maternal and neonatal mortality and morbidity in partnership with other stakeholders. In addition to their technical expertise, the status and social credibility of these professionals provide them with further opportunities to promote reproductive health and to positively influence health policy and practices in the field.

Their leadership lies in their ability to lobby, promote and educate the general public and governments about the essentials of health care for women, as well as to actively promote the collaborative approach among different groups of professionals involved in the delivery of healthcare for mother and their newborn [5]. They can also play an important role in advocating for changes in legislation and the development of policies in support of gender equality and the empowerment of women. Their potential contribution include:

- The development of national policies, strategies and action plans related to sexual and reproductive health, including maternal and newborn health;
- The strengthening and scaling up of health systems and health teams to enable them to provide effective low-cost interventions;
- The development and implementation of standards and protocols of care;
- The monitoring and evaluation of services to ensure quality care;
- The systematic review, through audits, of maternal mortalities and near-misses in order to identify their causes and implement actions to prevent their reoccurrence;
- The promotion of in-service and Continuing Medical Education (CME) programs for health professionals;
- The identification of social and cultural barriers affecting access of women to health services and, the implementation of actions to overcome these barriers;
- The promotion of open discussions on controversial issues such as access to safe abortion care, adolescent friendly reproductive health services and elimination of harmful practices such a gender-based violence and female genital mutilation;
- Discussions and actions aimed at creating greater synergy and intersection between initiatives focused on the reduction of maternal mortality and morbidity and those related to other aspects of sexual and reproductive health such as the provision of family planning services and the prevention and treatment of sexually transmitted infections including HIV/AIDS.

Professional associations are increasingly recognized as key partners for the reduction of maternal mortality and morbidity. Since the early 90's, ICM and FIGO have progressively increased their participation in global initiatives to reduce maternal and neonatal mortality and morbidity. Since 1987, ICM has been conducting workshops, usually as pre-congress activities, that bring together practitioners from countries with high rates of maternal mortality in an effort to provide them with comprehensive, up-to-date knowledge for making pregnancy and childbirth safer [6]. Similarly, in 1999, FIGO launched their first Save the Mothers Initiative, which consisted of the pairing of professional associations for projects in five lower income areas: Central America, Ethiopia, Mozambique, Pakistan and Uganda. The results of the projects demonstrated that "by motivating health professionals in the field and for a relatively modest financial outlay, more efficient use of existing services could be made in a sustainable fashion to save lives" [7]. Building on the experience acquired through this first generation of national projects, FIGO launched their Saving Mothers and Newborns Project in 2005. Finally, within this period, FIGO and ICM also collaborated on the development and dissemination of several joint policy statements addressing the critical role of skilled attendance during pregnancy and childbirth and the prevention of post partum hemorrhage through active management of the third stage of labor.

At national level, professional associations are also assuming leadership. For example, since 2003, professional associations from countries with high numbers of maternal deaths have been involved in national initiatives that seek to prevent and treat post partum hemorrhage. Supported by the Prevention of Postpartum Hemorrhage Initiative (POPPHI), a USAID funded global initiative, professional associations, both obstetricians/gynaecologists and midwives, are involved in expanding the use of Active Management of the Third Stage of Labour (AMSTL) in their respective countries [8]. Likewise, in 2005, the Ethiopian Society of Obstetricians and Gynaecologists launched a three-year initiative aimed at improving reproductive health services in three selected sites. Funded by the Packard Foundation, the project focuses on strengthening emergency obstetric care, increasing research on family planning and increasing advocacy for sexual and reproductive rights at the national level [9].

BUILDING CAPACITY OF PROFESSIONAL ASSOCIATIONS

In the early 1990s, the SOGC members initiated discussions and activities which eventually led to the establishment of its International Women's Health Program. This initial involvement in the international arena was linked to FIGO's growing commitment to promote safe motherhood and newborn health globally which gained momentum when FIGO held its XVI World Congress in Montreal, Canada in 1994.

In 1995, SOGC committed to promote international women's health by establishing an International Women's Health Committee and by initiating discussions with partners in lower resource countries for the conduct of joint initiatives. By 1998, SOGC formalized this commitment by recognizing, within its mission statement, the importance of pursuing excellence in international women's health and working toward the reduction of maternal mortality and morbidity worldwide. In the same year, the SOGC was successful in obtaining its first grant from CIDA for a two-year partnership initiative. This first experience laid the foundation for the SOGC's current capacity building partnership programs with Guatemala, Haiti and Uganda. In 1998, the SOGC also conducted in Uganda, in collaboration with the AOGU, a district intervention focusing on emergency obstetric care. These two initiatives led the Society, in 1999, to allocate the resources necessary for the establishment of its International Women's Health Program. Finally, SOGC has since reiterated this commitment by designating as a pillar, in its subsequent strategic plans, international women's health.

The SOGC's current international initiatives focus on: (a) increasing capacity of obstetricians/gynaecologists associations to promote maternal and neonatal care; (b) mobilizing and strengthening capacity of health professionals involved in the delivery of emergency obstetric care; and (c) increasing access, quality and utilization of emergency obstetric care at the level of the health system, through interventions at the community, health care delivery and referral levels.

The SOGC is also active in advocacy work related to sexual and reproductive health and rights, and more specifically safe motherhood and newborn health, at the international and national levels. In the international arena, Dr. Dorothy Shaw (SOGC President in 1991-1992 and currently FIGO President Elect) assumed, in 2000, the role of co-chair of the FIGO committee responsible for the development and implementation of its code of ethics related to sexual and reproductive health. In addition, in 2003, Dr. André Lalonde (SOGC Executive Vice President) was named co-chair of the FIGO Safe Motherhood and Newborn Health Committee. He further supported Dr. Arnoldo Acosta (FIGO past President) in the promotion of the Federation's global campaign calling for the prevention and treatment of post partum haemorrhage which was launched at the XVIII World Congress in Santiago, Chili in 2003. Dr Lalonde currently represents FIGO on the Coordinating Committee of the Partnership for Maternal, Newborn and Child Health, a global partnership bringing together leaders and advocates in developing and donor countries and working to mobilize global and local commitment and action to reduce maternal, newborn and child deaths in 60 high-burden countries [10].

Within Canada, the SOGC is also involved in advocacy for the increased role of Canada in promoting the right of women to survive pregnancy and childbirth worldwide. Since 2003, it published and disseminated several position papers calling on Canada to increase its investment in safe motherhood and newborn health, two of which were presented to the House of Commons' Standing Committee on Finance in October 2005 and September 2006 respectively

The international work of the SOGC is supported by two committees, the International Women's Health Committee and ALARM International Committee, which provide technical expertise on clinical and programmatic matters related to maternal and newborn health. Furthermore, the international work of the Society is sustained by a group of approximately 250 volunteer members, obstetricians/gynaecologists, general practitioners, midwives and nurses, interested in contributing their professional time and technical expertise in maternal and newborn health. Since 1999, the Society has conducted 77 interventions, in more than 14 countries, involving more than 140 volunteer opportunities.

Within its international program, the SOGC promotes the Programme of Action of the International Conference on Population and Development (ICPD) held in Cairo, Egypt in 1994 which defines reproductive health as follows:

"[…] a state of complete physical, mental and social well-being in all matters relating to the reproductive system and to its functions and processes. It implies that people have the capability to reproduce and the freedom to decide if, when and how often to do so. Implicit in this is the right of men and women to be informed and to have access to safe, effective, affordable and acceptable methods of family planning of their choice, as well as other methods of their choice for regulation of fertility, which are not against the law, and the right of access to health-care services that will enable women to go safely through pregnancy and childbirth [11]".

The international work of the SOGC is further guided by the following principles:

1. Safe motherhood is a basic human right and thus, ensuring safe motherhood and newborn health, is a matter of social justice;
2. Women's empowerment is a prerequisite for improved sexual and reproductive rights;
3. Women's poor sexual and reproductive health is influenced by a number of socioeconomic and cultural factors, all of which need to be addressed in order to improve women's health;
4. Safe motherhood and improved sexual and reproductive health can be achieved through access to quality basic health care;
5. Increasing access and utilization of skilled attendance at birth, including timely access to emergency obstetric care and the reduction of the three delays to emergency obstetric care (delays in deciding to seek care, in identifying and reaching medical facility and in receiving the adequate and appropriate medical treatment once at the health facility) are critical interventions to reduce maternal mortality and morbidity;

6. Health professionals and by extension, their professional associations, obstetricians, general practitioners, midwives and nurses, have an important role to play in not only ensuring women's access to quality sexual and reproductive health services but also respecting and promoting women's sexual and reproductive rights;

7. Partnerships, between professional associations from higher and lower income countries, multi and bilateral institutions, organizations or non-governmental organizations (NGOs) and others, are viable and sustainable means to promote global, regional and national safe motherhood and newborn health;

8. Monitoring and evaluation are core components for all international initiatives led by health professionals. [12]

PARTNERSHIP MODEL OF SOGC

SOGC's capacity building work with professional associations is based on the premise that strong and vibrant professional associations can play an important role in the promotion of women's reproductive health and rights, including the reduction of maternal and neonatal mortality and morbidity. The Society also believes that partnerships, between professional associations from lower and higher resource countries, are viable and sustainable means by which to promote safer pregnancy and childbirth.

Within its international partnership initiatives, SOGC shares with its partners the Society's knowledge, technical expertise, skills and experiences which have contributed to its own capacity to build a strong and credible national association that can influence national policy and to contribute to the improvement of women's health outcomes in Canada. It further shares the clinical and programmatic knowledge and expertise acquired through its involvement in the global safe motherhood and newborn health movement.

The Society's work with professional associations is also guided by its strong commitment to promote a participatory approach within all of its partnership relationships. This approach ensures ample opportunity for all partners to contribute their expertise and knowledge, and to apply their newly developed leadership capacity as the partnership relationship progresses. The Society's main role is thus seen as a catalyst, in which society members provide technical expertise as mentors, facilitators, trainers, coaches and expert counsels.

The experience acquired by SOGC within its partnership programs confirms that professional associations from lower income countries have the interest, will and the commitment to promote safe motherhood and newborn health globally and nationally, and that when provided with appropriate support and guidance, can acquire the capacity to do so. Furthermore, a recent evaluation of the partnership program of the Society confirms that organizational capacity can be strengthened with modest resources. To date, within its partnership program with the professional associations of Guatemala, Haiti and Uganda, approximately 56,000 USD per year per association proved sufficient to yield positive results in enhancing the organizational capacity of each association [13].

BUILDING CAPACITY AT COUNTRY LEVEL

"We have had more activities in the last 3 years than in the past 47 years in the life of the association."

SHOG (Haiti)

"We moved from being an association involved in social and cultural activities to one involved in activities resulting in social change."

AGOG (Guatemala)

"The partnership program provided the association with an opportunity to diversify its activities and contribute to more practical and technical issues."

AOGU (Uganda) [14]

The SOGC has been involved since 1998 in capacity building partnerships with AGOG from Guatemala, SHOG from Haiti and AOGU from Uganda. SOGC's work in all three countries has been supported by CIDA, through two project cycles (1998/1999 and 1999/2002) and one three-year program cycle which was renewed in January 2007. The partnership initiatives focus on strengthening the organizational capacities of partner associations to increase their leadership in the promotion of women's reproductive health and rights, with a focus on safe motherhood and newborn health. The main objectives of the partnership initiatives include: (a) strengthening the capacities of partner associations with regard to structure, self-governance and management practices; (b) enhancing their technical and programmatic expertise with regard to low cost interventions related to the reduction of maternal mortality and morbidity; and finally (c) building knowledge and skills with regard to the promotion of the sexual and reproductive rights based approach as it applies to maternal and infant health.

The activities and support provided to partner associations consist of:

- Financial support and technical assistance for the establishment or upgrade of national secretariats, including support for new communication technologies (e.g. internet and email);
- Training and technical assistance related to program management practices, including the Results-Based Management (RBM) approach and gender sensitivity;
- Financial and technical support for the development, implementation and evaluation of strategic plans;
- Production and dissemination of Information, Education and Communication (IEC) material related to women's sexual and reproductive health and rights;
- Train-the-trainers programs for the establishment of a national pool of ALARM International Program instructors in the countries of intervention;
- Provision of the ALARM International Program's training curriculum and other educational materials and supplies necessary to deliver the program;
- Financial support and technical assistance for in-country initiatives, primarily related to the delivery of the ALARM International Program;

- Support to facilitate partner participation at international technical meetings or forums promoting cost-effective interventions and/or strategies related to maternal and infant health;
- Study tours and partnership meetings in Canada;
- Technical assistance and support for in-country workshops/seminars related to making pregnancy and childbirth safer, most of them conducted within the partners' annual scientific meetings.

A review of the experience and the outcomes of the partnership program, for both partner associations and SOGC, are positive and promising. They confirm the interest and commitment of professional associations to assume leadership in the promotion of safer pregnancy and childbirth, especially in their respective countries. These experiences also provide greater insight and better understanding of the factors that contribute or limit the participation of professional associations in initiatives aimed at reducing maternal and neonatal mortality and morbidity.

Overall, the main outcomes of the CIDA-funded partnership have been: increased capacity of partner associations to manage expanded programs and activities of their associations, participation and contribution of partners in national initiatives aimed at reducing maternal deaths and injuries, and increased collaboration with other stakeholders involved in the field of safe motherhood and newborn health.

INCREASING ORGANIZATIONAL CAPACITY

The partnership with SOGC led all partner associations to upgrade the capacity of their national secretariats in order to better support and manage their expanding programs and activities, including services to members. All partners proved able to recruit core staff for their secretariats and, to open their offices to members during regular office hours. For example, both AOGU and SHOG made their high speed internet services available to members thereby allowing them to communicate with peers internationally and to access the growing number of evidence-based resources made available on the web by major stakeholders in the field (such as WHO, UNFPA and JHPIEGO). All three associations further developed knowledge and skills related to the planning, implementation, monitoring and reporting of programs and projects. These skills provided them with the capacity to respond to calls for proposals for in-country health initiatives. For example, both SHOG and AOGU responded to a call for proposals from FIGO for the Saving Mothers and Newborns Project, and successfully submitted projects aiming the improvement of obstetric care in selected districts of their respective countries.

With the support of the SOGC, the partner associations revised their organizational structures and completed strategic plans in order to enhance their capacity to respond to the country's health needs. The strategic planning exercises led the associations to revise their mission statements to better reflect their expanded role in the promotion of women's health. It also led them to modify their by-laws for the purpose of broadening their memberships to include allied health professionals and to facilitate the participation of different categories of members. For example, in Uganda, a representative from the community serves on the

Executive Committee of the association. In an effort to promote the collaborative approach, all partners implemented a strategy to increase the participation of other allied health professionals, members and non members, in the programs of the associations, including CME activities. These actions resulted in increased and more diversified memberships, increased services to members, increased number of members involved in the programs and activities of the associations, improved program management practices and programs that are better aligned to the health needs of each country.

ENHANCING CONTRIBUTION AT NATIONAL LEVEL

Strengthening technical and programmatic capacity of professionals associations in safe motherhood and newborn health programs was done, from the beginning of the partnership initiatives, through the SOGC's ALARM International Program, an internationally recognized mobilizing and capacity building tool for health professionals involved in the delivery of emergency obstetric care. The program is endorsed by FIGO, and is recognized by WHO as an effective tool for the dissemination of the guidelines and practices outlined in its reference manual: *Managing Complications in Pregnancy and Childbirth: A Guide for Midwives and Doctors* [15]. The ALARM International Program focuses its education and practice on the five main causes of maternal mortality and morbidity, initiates discussion and activities for integrating the sexual and reproductive rights approach to safe motherhood and newborn health programs, and further builds capacity with regard to maternal mortality audit methodologies. A module on newborn care, including newborn resuscitation, was integrated into the program with the support of the Canadian Paediatric Society and Saving Newborns Lives in 2003.

The ALARM International Program was developed and piloted, by the Society through its current partnership program with AGOG, AOGU and SHOG. Since 1999, the ALARM International Program training component has been offered in several other countries with high rates of maternal deaths, including Gabon, India, Indonesia, Mali, Mexico, the Philippines, Zambia, and Yemen. Designed originally for the purpose of either a CME or in-service training, the ALARM International Program is being expanded and modified into a series of educational activities, spread over a 3-year period, for health professionals involved in obstetrics.

Within the SOGC partnership initiatives, all three partner associations have developed the capacity to promote the ALARM International Program with little support from the SOGC. Using the train-the-trainers approach, national teams of ALARM International Instructors were established in all three countries of intervention. Furthermore, all associations were provided with the program's curriculum and the accompanying educational equipment, materials and supplies (such as lap top computers, LCD projectors, obstetrical mannequins, neonatal dolls and forceps) necessary for the delivery of the training component of the program. The partners were also exposed to new cost-effective interventions in the field through their participation in capacity building initiatives in Canada (such as the annual partnership program meeting) and through other international forums, such as the pre congress workshops of the FIGO World Congresses in both Santiago, Chili and Kuala

Lumpur, Malaysia and a technical workshop on maternal audits offered by WHO's within its *Beyond the Numbers* initiative [16]. .

All partners have integrated the ALARM International Program to the annual program of activities of their association. Additionally, in partnership with other stakeholders, partner associations have conducted the training component of ALARM International Program within specific maternal and newborn health initiatives in their respective countries. From 2003-2006, AGOG in Guatemala conducted the ALARM International Program within 16 ministry-led initiatives in priority districts of the country. Likewise in Uganda, AOGU offered the program in a community initiative conducted by a national NGO involved in the area of HIV/AIDS. Finally, SHOG in Haiti conduted the program within a UNICEF/UNFPA maternal health initiative conducted in three priority departments of the country. SHOG proved successful in building in their intiative a pre training needs assessment and support supervision activities after the training activities. The initiatives in all three countries were supported by a number of international health organizations and donors.

Within the recently completed partnership phase (2003/06), AGOG and AOGU further opted to direct their technical capacities toward the implementation of the ALARM International Program in selected health districts of their respective countries. Within both district interventions (Chimaltenango, Guatemala and Masaka, Uganda), the national partner associations upgraded the skills of health professionals in emergency obstetric care and provided support supervision activities. Furthermore, the associations offered technical assistance to the districts with regard to maternal audits, standards of care, clinical guidelines and strategies to strengthen links with the community. Although these specific initiatives remain to be evaluated, preliminary information confirms the capacity of these professional associations to expand their leadership role beyond trainers in CME types of activities, to one of collaborators and technical experts in initiatives aiming to strengthen the capacities of health centers and health teams to provide quality emergency obstetric care.

The knowledge, skills, programmatic expertise and experience gained through the building of capacity with regard to the ALARM International Program has also enabled the professional associations to expand their proficiency in the field of maternal and infant health. In Guatemala, AGOG used the content of the ALARM International Program in the development of national guidelines and protocols related to emergency obstetric care. In Haiti, SHOG borrowed modules and methodologies from the ALARM International Program to educate residents about emergency obstetric care. And finally, in Uganda, AOGU applied the information within the women's sexual and reproductive health and rights module of the program to conduct community mobilization activities in selected districts of the country.

Since 1998, the role of SOGC has evolved from trainer to mentor. The Society now focuses its intervention on enhancing the capacity of the associations to promote the ALARM International Program to other key actors within their respective countries. It also supports activities that intend to keep the partners updated on evidence-based practices and cost-effective innovations in obstetrics and enhance their competency related to the methodology of the ALARM International Program.

INCREASING COLLABORATION WITH INTERNATIONAL AND NATIONAL STAKEHOLDERS

The partnership initiatives resulted in the ability of all the partners to strengthen their relationships with other stakeholders in the field, whether at the international, national, regional or local levels. All partner associations developed strong collaborative links with the national health ministries of their countries, and other multilateral agencies and institutions involved in the health sector. Additionally, all partners established or strengthened partnership links with universities, research institutions and other NGOs involved in maternal and newborn health. The associations also increased their involvement in community level activities by either involving themselves in community mobilizing activities or initiating actions aimed at identifying identify and acting upon barriers to care.

The type and quality of partnerships that have developed over the years are diverse. The following represent a few examples. In Uganda, AOGU is exploring ways to better support women choosing traditional birthing positions during labour and delivery at health centers as a way to improve women's perception of quality care and to decrease the barriers to skilled attendance. In Haiti, SHOG conducted workshops at the national nurse-midwifery school to promote the use of vacuum extraction for assisted deliveries. And finally, in Guatemala, AGOG collaborated with other national stakeholders for the dissemination of the findings of a national study on gender-based violence.

LESSONS LEARNED

After almost ten years of work and experience in supporting professional associations in strengthening their capacities to assume leadership in the field of women's health, SOGC has learned the following lessons and subsequently established the following best practices.

Lessons Learned

- Obstetricians/gynaecologists are key stakeholders in the global movement calling for the reduction of maternal and newborn mortality and morbidity. Their commitment to safe motherhood and newborn health is supported by their increasing involvement in global and national efforts promoting cost-effective interventions and strategies in the field.
- Strong and vibrant professional associations are capable of promoting sexual and reproductive health and rights, including women's right to survive pregnancy and childbirth. Their leadership can positively contribute to the implementation, monitoring and evaluation of sustainable national maternal and newborn health programs aimed at reducing maternal and neonatal mortality and morbidity.
- Professional associations require strong organizational capacity to expand their programs, influence policy and contribute to international and national efforts in the field of safe motherhood and newborn health. Strong organizational capacity permits

associations to undertake their activities in a planned and sustainable manner in order to better respond to the health needs of their countries.

- Building capacity of professional associations to increase their involvement in the promotion of women's health takes time and resources. SOGC's experience shows that for greatest impact and sustainability, a commitment of 8 to10 years of support is needed.

- Members of professional associations can be mobilized to contribute, as volunteers, to national and regional (within the country) safe motherhood and newborn health activities and programs. SOGC member volunteers contributed more than 500,000 USD of in-kind professional time within the 2003-2006 partnership program.

Best Practices

- Facilitating the participation of professional associations from lower resource countries to global forums (such as conferences and technical meetings sponsored by FIGO, WHO, the Partnership for Maternal, Newborn and Child Health) enhances their commitment and their capacity to contribute to safe motherhood and newborn health efforts. Participation at these forums provides them with opportunities to:
    - o Network and exchange information and experience with health experts from around the world;
    - o Remain updated on tools, new cost-effective interventions, best practices and policies;
    - o Increase their knowledge and understanding of the multilateral institutions' global and national strategies which directly impact the organization and the delivery of health services in their countries (such as Sector Wide Approach Programs and Poverty Reduction Strategy Papers);
    - o Establish regional partnerships with other stakeholders;
    - o Facilitate the linkages with national government and multilateral agency representatives from their respective countries.
- The ALARM International Program is an educational and mobilizing tool with great potential in global and national efforts to strengthen health systems, especially with regards to increasing competency of the skills of health professionals and increasing capacity of health systems.
- Building capacity of professional associations to promote the ALARM International Program has proven to be a successful means by which to strengthen their overall organizational capacities, including enhancing their credibility and expertise in other maternal mortality and morbidity related interventions, such as monitoring and evaluation of maternal deaths and near-misses and the development of national guidelines and protocols.
- The train-the-trainers approach is a viable and successful methodology for the transfer of knowledge and skills with regard to the ALARM International Program.
- Promoting safe motherhood and newborn health using the human rights approach is needed to truly impact on the high rates of maternal mortality and morbidity globally and to work toward women's empowerment.

- Partnership initiatives between professional associations from higher and lower resource countries are innovative ways to ensure the transfer of knowledge and capacity through the exchange of technical expertise and experience between them.

CLOSING WORDS

"It is not enough to be clinically competent. It is not enough to be socially aware and socially conscious. The obstetrician and gynaecologist must be a champion for ALL women's health, welfare and rights [...] (they) must become the voices of the voiceless, the champions of the neglected, the militants of the poor. Their leadership and their social and economic clout are needed to make essential obstetric care available to all women. Their actions and voices are necessary to shift resources at the national level [...] to improve [...] health systems. It is time [...] to move beyond the consulting room, beyond the hospital ward, to play a prominent part in the revitalization of the health system as a whole."

Dr. T. Türmen, WHO (2000) [17]

SOGC's involvement in the international arena, has been exciting and invigorating not only for the Society as a whole, but for its members and staff, especially those most implicated in the Society's International Women's Health Program. It has provided the Society and its members an opportunity to put into practice, at the international level, its philosophy and practices related to the strength and value of partnerships for the advancement of women's health. The program has also provided an opportunity for them to acquire knowledge, experience and skills pertaining to policies and practices aimed at reducing maternal and neonatal mortality and morbidity. For these reasons, it remains ever thankful to its longest standing partners, the *Asociacion de Gynecologia y Obstetricia de Guatemala* (AGOG), the Association of Obstetricians and Gynaecologists of Uganda (UAOG) and last but not least, *la Société Haïtienne d'Obstétrique et de Gynécologie*.

The achievements of the partnership program of the Society confirms the commitment and capacity of professional associations, from lower and higher resource countries, to assess, plan, initiate and commit themselves to the promotion of safe motherhood and newborn health. Their contribution can increase significantly in the next decade, provided that the international community carries out their commitment to increase resources and polical will to achieve the Millennium Development Goals related to maternal and newborn health. Within this call to action, professional associations, especially those from the countries most concerned, are well positioned to assume leadership in national efforts aimed at strengthening the capacities of health systems to ensure safer pregnancies and childbirth, especially with regard to emergency obstetric care. As SOGC's experience clearly demonstrates, their ability to assume this leadership role is critical to the building of strong and vibrant associations capable of responding to the health needs of their countries. The challenge is thus in finding innovative ways to support these professional associations so that they can develop the ability to assume this leadership role. Partnership initiatives between professional associations from higher and lower resource countries are one such innovation.

Finally, SOGC challenges international and national leaders and advocates to foster opportunities for professional associations from lower resource countries to strengthen their capacity and to join the global movement for safe motherhood and newborn health.

Supporting capacity building initiatives of professional associations, including partnership programs of professional associations between higher and lower resource countries, are progressive and sustainable means to ensure the full participation of these key stakeholders in the international and national efforts to improve maternal and infant health, and consequently to have a positive impact on the unacceptable high rates of maternal and neonatal mortality and morbidity which persist in many parts of the world.

REFERENCES

[1]   Fathalla M. Safe motherhood: an inter-agency challenge [oral presentation]. World Health Day. Safe motherhood: progress and challenges; 1998 Apr 7; Washington. Available: *http://www.safemotherhood.org/SMat10/world_health_day/mahmoud_fat halla.htm* (accessed 2007 Jan 11).

[2]   Facts and figures from the World Health Report. Geneva: World Health Organization; 2005. Available: *http://www.who.int/whr/2005/media_centre/facts_en.pdf* (accessed 2007 Nov 1).

[3]   Best Practices Sub-committee, White Ribbon Alliance for Safe Motherhood/India. Saving mothers' lives - what works: a field guide for implementing best practices in safe motherhood. New Delhi: The Alliance; 2002. Available: *http://www.cedpa.org /content/publication/detail/744* (accessed 2007 Jan 11).

[4]   Making pregnancy safer: the critical role of the skilled attendant. A joint statement by WHO, ICM and FIGO. Geneva: World Health Organization; 2004. Available: *http://www.who.int/reproductive-health/publications/2004/skilled_attendant.pdf* (accessed 2007 Jan 11).

[5]   Chamberlain J, McDonagh R, Lalonde A, Arulkumaran S. The role of professional associations in reducing maternal mortality worldwide. *Int J Gynaecol Obset* 2003;83(1):94-102.

[6]   ICM Collaborative Safe Motherhood workshop, July 21-23: 'Promoting the Health of Mothers and Newborns during Birth and the Postnatal Period' [news release]. The Hague: International Confederation of Midwives; 2005 Jul 23. Available: *http://www.medicalknowledgeinstitute.com/files/Safe%20Motherhood%20workshop%2 0Brisbane%202005.pdf* (accessed 2007 Jan 3).

[7]   Benagiano G, Thomas B. Safe motherhood: the FIGO initiative. *Int J Gynaecol Obstet* 2003;82(3):263-74.

[8]   Prevention of Postpartum Hemorrhage Initiative. Small grants. Washington: The Initiative; 2006. Available*: http://www.pphprevention.org/small_grants.php* (accessed 2007 Jan 5).

[9]   Projects. Addis Ababa: Ethiopian Society of Obstetricians and Gynecologists; 2007. Available: *http://www.esog.org.et/Projects.htm* (accessed 2007 Jan 3).

[10]   Partnership for Maternal, Newborn & Child Health. What we do. Geneva: World Health Organization; 2007. Available: *http://www.who.int/pmnch/activities/en/* (accessed 2007 Jan 5).

[11] Summary of the ICPD Programme of Action. New York: United Nations; 1995.
      DPI/1618/POP. Available: *http://www.unfpa.org/icpd/summary.htm* (accessed 2007 Jan
      11).

[12] Framework for international policy initiatives [policy statement]. Ottawa: Society of
      Obstetricians and Gynaecologists of Canada; 2005 Mar. Available: *http://sogc.medical.*
      org/iwhp/pdf/IWH-framework_e.pdf (accessed 2007 Jan 11).

[13] *SOGC Partnership Program (1998 - 2006): assessment of organization capacity for*
      long-term benefits. Ottawa: DS Bateson Consulting Inc.; 2006 Aug 29.

[14] *SOGC Partnership Program 2003-2006: Partnership meeting report May 23rd to 29th,*
      2003 - Ottawa, Canada. Ottawa: Society of Obstetricians and Gynaecologists of
      Canada; 2003.

[15] Department of Reproductive Health and Childbirth, Family and Community Health,
      World Health Organization. Managing complications in pregnancy and childbirth: a
      guide for midwives and doctors [Intergrated management of pregnancy and childbirth].
      Geneva: The Organization; 2003. WHO/RHR/00.7. Available*: http://www.who.int/*
      reproductive-health/impac/mcpc.pdf (accessed 2007 Jan 11).

[16] World Health Organization. Beyond numbers: reviewing maternal deaths and
      complications to make pregnancy safer. Geneva: The Organization; 2004. Available:
      http://www.who.int/reproductive-health/publications/btn/text.pdf (accessed 2007 Jan
      11).

[17] Türmen T. Emergency obstetric care for all women - a social responsibility for
      obstetricians [workshop]. XVII FIGO World Congress; 2000 Aug; Washington.

In: Women's Health in the Majority World: Issues and Initiatives   ISBN1-1-60021-493-2
Eds: L. Elit and J. Chamberlain Froese, pp. 155-178   © 2007 Nova Science Publishers, Inc.

Chapter 9

THE ROLE OF NONGOVERNMENTAL ORGANIZATIONS IN PROMOTING WOMEN'S HEALTH IN LOW-RESOURCE SETTINGS

Patricia S. Coffey[1], Allison Bingham,
Harriet Stanley, and John W. Sellors
PATH, 1455 NW Leary Way, Seattle, WA 98107, U.S.A.

ABSTRACT

Nongovernmental organizations (NGOs) are typically value-based organizations that depend, in whole or in part, on charitable donations and voluntary service. Although the NGO sector has become increasingly professionalized over the last two decades, it is generally recognized that principles of altruism and voluntarism still remain key defining characteristics.

In this chapter, various definitions of the NGO will be introduced and discussed, including those offered by the World Bank and theWorld Health Organization. A literature review related to the evolving nature of NGO involvement in advancing women's health in the 20th and 21st centuries also will be undertaken. In the review, the authors emphasize the role of NGOs in health service delivery, health promotion, and policy advocacy related to women's health. They also review the evolving participation of international NGOs in initiating and contributing to global health policy and highlight global trends in NGO involvement in women's health.

The following section envisions a future for NGOs. Important questions related to their role in low-resource settings in the 21st century are delineated. The chapter then explores the key challenges and opportunities for NGOs to address women's health issues. Key challenges include organizational growth and development, assessing and strengthening performance, sustainability, representation and accountability, politicized foreign assistance, religious fundamentalism and human rights. Key opportunities include collaboration with the private sector, the community and government, and reconfiguring reliance on international assistance. The section offers examples of cutting edge NGOs in

---

[1] Contact: Dr. Patricia S.Coffey: PATH, 1455 NW Leary Way, Seattle, WA 98107,email: *pcoffey@path.org;* tel: 206.285-3500.

action and draws from lessons learned by PATH and other international NGOs. PATH is discussed as an example of a specific NGO model that emphasizes collaboration between governments, local NGOs, civil society, and corporate business communities through institutional partnerships. Examples of specific program outcomes illustrate how this model functions successfully.

INTRODUCTION

Nongovernmental organizations (NGOs) have emerged as major players in global development, particularly in the health sector. In 2006, the *Directory of Development Organizations* listed more than 47,500 organizations devoted to international development worldwide [1]. One can easily access more than 51,000 nonprofit and community organizations in 165 countries on the Internet, and the list grows daily [2].

The number and diversity of NGOs is particularly apparent in the health and social-services sectors. In the health sector, the number of international NGOs grew from 1,357 to 2,036 from 1990 to 2000 [3]. The growth of NGOs working in the social services sector has been even more substantial.

This proliferation of NGOs has been accompanied by a growing body of literature on the role and effectiveness of NGOs in all sectors. This chapter will discuss the evolving definition and nature of NGOs and the role they play in promoting women's health, particularly in service provision, promotion of positive behaviors, and policy advocacy. The authors explore the internal and external factors that constrain or enhance NGOs' potential for addressing women's health and, by examining profiles of NGOs in action, they highlight principles that are key to successful NGO activities in low-resource settings.

WHAT IS AN NGO?

NGOs are typically described as value-based or mission-driven organizations that depend, in whole or in part, on charitable donations and voluntary service [4]. They are classified as nonprofit organizations. While some researchers note that no single definition of NGOs is broadly accepted [5], certain features figure prominently. For example:

NGOs are generally independent from the direct control of government.

- They do not act as a political party.
- They are nonprofit.
- They do not engage in criminal activities.

Willetts describes NGOs as "independent voluntary association[s] of people acting together on a continuous basis, for some common purpose, other than achieving government office, making money or illegal activities [5]." The World Bank uses a more specific definition, describing NGOs as "private organizations that pursue activities to relieve suffering, promote the interests of the poor, protect the environment, provide basic social services, or undertake community development [6]."

As these descriptions imply, voluntarism and altruism are often thought to be the defining characteristics of NGOs [6]. In our experience, the NGO community is becoming increasingly diverse and now reflects a range of approaches including some NGOs that feature highly paid professional staff.

How are NGOs Structured?

NGOs are structured in a variety of ways. They can be organized at the local, regional, national, or international levels. A common model of an NGO is an organization in which individuals work in local groups, with coordination coming from the provincial or national level and the headquarters based in a capital city.

Individuals can become involved with NGOs through employment as paid staff or by joining as supportive members. NGO members who contribute volunteer labor are usually among the intended beneficiaries of the organization's efforts. Most NGOs are membership organizations, meaning that individuals support the organization through volunteer labor, financial assistance, or both. NGOs range in size and focus from small, community-oriented NGOs to large and well-established international NGOs such as Oxfam, Red Cross International, and ActionAid.

CBOs, CSOs, and PVOs

Grassroots organizations that are locally based are sometimes referred to as community-based organizations, or CBOs. Recently, CBOs have been included as an important component of a broader concept that the World Health Organization (WHO) has defined: civil society organizations, or CSOs [7,8]. According to WHO, "individuals and groups organize themselves into CSOs to pursue their collective interests and engage in activities of public importance [9]." CSOs are non-state, nonprofit, voluntary organizations that may or may not link to the market or state. CSO membership generally goes beyond immediate family ties and includes individuals from extended social networks such as neighborhoods, community, work, or social networks.

The distinction between NGOs and CSOs denotes the fact that, in many countries, NGOs retain a formal structure and are required to register with national authorities. CSOs, on the other hand, are not required to register with the government, although they do provide an avenue for individuals to interact in a collective manner with government or commercial institutions. In the United States, NGOs that solicit and receive cash contributions from the general public are often referred to as private voluntary organizations, or PVOs.

Throughout this chapter, the term "NGO" is used to refer to this range of organizations, including CBOs, CSOs, PVOs, and other variations.

Local and Regional NGOs

Local and regional NGOs are molded by the geographical, sociocultural, political, and economic realities of where they work. To effectively collaborate with a local NGO, it is essential to understand the organizational context and goals. Locally run, community-based organizations that organize themselves around funding opportunities tend to fit the traditional description of organizations that are based on altruism or volunteerism. They often are created in response to a recurring issue or problem that impacts the quality of life in their community (e.g., lack of a clean water supply or low literacy levels) or to pursue broadly defined and conceptual outcomes such as "increasing women's empowerment." In resource-poor settings, they may lack technical capacity, political influence, the ability to organize and work with others, or an adequate resource base to implement long-lasting improvements. In our experience, membership-based NGOs form a distinct sub-group that must address member needs while, at the same time, focus on project outcomes. This competition for organizational focus may result in a more limited capacity to deliver measurable project outcomes than other NGOs. While the workers are certainly more aware of grassroots issues and cultural nuances, they may have difficulty proving impact of an intervention. Increasingly, however, NGOs are becoming more professional in their approaches and more rigorous in their monitoring and evaluation efforts.

International and Transnational NGOs

International NGOs reach across borders to attract members and supporters motivated by a particular cause or area of concern that the organization embraces as its reason to exist.

Many of the larger, international NGOs such as the International Planned Parenthood Federation (www.ippf.org) and CARE International (www.care.org) also fit the definition of transnational NGOs. These NGOs, which generally are membership organizations, provide a global forum where activist members may work to influence corporate activity or address inadequate performance of the state [10]. Transnational NGOs are supported by members and staff who want to create a more just world. In the health sector, many transnational NGOs, such as Development Alternatives for Women with a New Era, work to promote women and human rights [11].

The number of transnational NGOs is growing in step with today's expanding global economy. Like all NGOs, these transnational organizations function independently of government control and are nonprofit. The distinctive feature of transnational NGOs is their commitment to advocacy and their belief that they can significantly impact corporate activity and governmental policies. They work through specific campaigns directed toward their vision of universal human rights protection, conflict resolution, and environmental preservation [10]. In this regard, they operate across borders to impact public causes, and many have leaders from a variety of cultural and national backgrounds [12].

WHAT IS THE ROLE OF AN NGO?

The basic role of an NGO is to act as a bridge between the individual and the state. Most NGOs work in one of three general ways: they complement existing governmental and other institutions, they take positions that are critical of the government, or they are unofficially embedded in a governmental structure. Let's discuss each of these roles in more detail.

First and perhaps most important, NGOs may work in a complementary manner with existing governmental and other institutions. For example, NGOs sometimes partner with governments to enable them to strengthen their service capacity despite restrictive policies or difficult political environments. One way they can do this is to use pilot projects to introduce expanded services or new commodities without contravening existing policy. In an environment where it may be extremely difficult to change existing policies, this partnering offers opportunities for government staff to respond more quickly to the needs of their local population and to obtain locally relevant evidence on the safety and effectiveness of an intervention. This type of complementary action demonstrates the NGO's ability to identify and address gaps in services, advocate for solutions, and collaborate with government partners within the context of flexible policies.

Second, some NGOs may take positions that are critical of the government. So-called "activist" NGOs are often the most effective in giving a voice to marginalized groups. Some give voice in a relatively subtle manner, such as the Empower Foundation, a 20-year-old Thai NGO made up of thousands of sex workers. This group recently opened a drop-in center for sex workers in Phang Nga, a mountainous province on the Andaman Sea that was the epicenter of the 2004 tsunami. The NGO is providing relief to the local sex workers affected by the tsunami because they fall outside the labor law and are, therefore, not entitled to financial assistance from the government [13]. In doing so, they are both complementing the government's services and validating the needs of a population that the government tends to overlook.

Other NGOs are more directly confrontational in their strategies. For instance, in Zimbabwe, the Women and AIDS Support Network (WASN), an NGO comprised of community-based women's groups and associations, played a major role in persuading the government to add the female condom to the country's mix of available contraceptive methods. Initially, the government was hesitant about procuring the female condom because the method was not approved by their national regulatory agency. WASN leadership began a public campaign to demand the device's expeditious approval to ensure its commercial availability. To incorporate women's voices, WASN launched a petition drive that was promoted by an extensive media campaign. By World AIDS Day (December 1) 1996, 30,000 signatures had been collected through the efforts of WASN and other women's NGOs. In September 1996, Zimbabwe's Medical Control Council approved the female condom for use, largely as a result of this action. In July 1997, the government began delivering the device in both the public and private sectors [14].

Third, some NGOs are unofficially but functionally embedded in the governmental structure. In Africa, some women's NGOs act as an unofficial arm of a political party. In one East African country where we have worked, the local NGO partner used project monitoring visits to health centers and village sites as an opportunity to mobilize voter registration, especially among women's groups, and to recruit party members during election time. This aberration was viewed as an acceptable practice in the country, and it was understood that little project-related work would be carried out before the election.

How Are NGOs Helping to Advance Women's Health?

A 2002 literature review by WHO concluded that NGOs are contributing to global health in terms of technical expertise, community or social experiences, information for health systems, and institutional resources for health outreach.

Table 1. NGOs' roles in women's health.

Health system function	Possible NGO roles
Health service delivery	Provide family planning, reproductive, and sexual health services. Facilitate community interactions with services. Distribute health resources such as condoms or clean delivery kits. Build health worker morale and support.
Health promotion and information exchange	Obtain and disseminate health information about family planning and reproductive and sexual health provision. Build informed public choice by raising awareness about these options. Implement and use health research. Help shift social attitudes. Mobilize and organize for health.
Policy setting	Represent public and community interests in policy. Promote equity and pro-poor policies. Negotiate public health standards and approaches. Build policy consensus; disseminate policy positions. Enhance public support for policies.
Resource mobilization and allocation	Finance health services. Raise community preferences in resource allocation. Mobilize and organize community co-financing of services. Promote pro-poor and equity concerns in resource allocation. Build public accountability and transparency in raising, allocating, and managing resources.
Monitoring quality of care and responsiveness	Monitor responsiveness and quality of health services. Give voice to marginalized groups; promote equity. Represent patient rights in quality of care issues. Channel and negotiate patient complaints and claims.

Adapted from WHO/CSI: 2001 [9].

The authors found that NGO interventions appear to be more effective when social action, public advocacy, or innovative and community-based responses to health problems are used. In addition, the report cited evidence suggesting that NGOs' influence on global health policy is exerted primarily through the political force of networking, building alliances, creating linkages, advocacy, and other coalition-type activities [15].

A useful framework for examining the contributions of NGOs—or, more broadly speaking, civil society—to improving health systems was presented in a WHO paper [9]. We have adapted this framework to highlight five health systems functions and associated roles that NGOs can play in advancing women's health (table 1).

Next, we look at examples of how NGOs contribute to specific health system functions (mentioned above) that are aimed towards improving women's health.

Health Service Delivery

NGOs have long been involved in the delivery of health services in developing countries. For many years, NGOs have provided clinical care to many underserved or marginalized populations. In some cases, NGOs have filled a need that government was unable or unwilling to meet. At times this work has been conducted in close partnership with a government, as the NGO may deliver services and the government may monitor service quality (or vice versa). NGOs can also play a role in private-sector service delivery by providing training on new or underutilized technologies and best clinical practices.

Historically, the provision of family planning services has been viewed as a low priority by some governments, particularly in sub-Saharan Africa. To address this need, the International Planned Parenthood Federation (IPPF) began providing sexual and reproductive health services. IPPF built a member structure comprised of Family Planning Associations supported in 149 countries. The focus of IPPF work continues in five priority areas: adolescents, HIV/AIDS, abortion, access to services, and advocacy. In 2003, approximately 32 million visits were made to IPPF facilities. These visits resulted in more than 23.2 million cycles of oral pills and 102 million condoms being distributed, and 2.4 million people were newly introduced to family planning. Other services provided by IPPF facilities included counseling, gynecological care, HIV/AIDS-related activities, diagnosis and treatment of sexually transmitted infections (STIs), mother and child health, and abortion-related services.[2] The reach of these services illustrates the impact that an NGO can have on health service delivery.

Health Promotion

Health promotion refers to developing awareness of health needs and interventions, encouraging healthy behaviors, and supporting environments that are conducive to good health practices. The promotion of reproductive and sexual health using a variety of communication materials often accompanies service-delivery initiatives implemented by NGOs. For example, the Media/Materials Clearinghouse, which is maintained by the Center for Communication Programs at the Johns Hopkins University Bloomberg School of Public Health, features health communication materials from around the world. This international resource is available online (http://www.m-mc.org) and distributes a range of health communication materials: pamphlets, posters, audiotapes, videos, training materials, job aids, electronic media, and other materials designed to promote public health.

Social Marketing

Social marketing is another health promotion method that is often used by NGOs in low-resource settings. Social marketing uses the same marketing principles and psychosocial

---

[2] International Planned Parenthood website. Available at: *www.ippf.org.* Accessed February 22, 2006.

theories that are used to sell products to consumers by changing their perceptions, attitudes, and behaviors. This technique has been used extensively in international health programs, particularly to raise awareness and change behavior related to contraception—including products and services such as male and female condoms, oral contraceptives, IUDs, injectable contraceptives, emergency contraceptive pills, voluntary surgical contraception, pregnancy test kits, and clean delivery kits [17].

Interactive Media

Another innovative way to raise awareness about important sexual and reproductive health issues is through interactive community theater performances. PATH, an international NGO, pioneered an approach called "Magnet Theater" due to the natural "pulling" power of theater to engage audiences in a participatory manner. Experience has shown that when theater performances occur regularly in the same location over time, community members are attracted in increasing numbers to join the dialogue and to participate in performances based on their local situation and issues. In Bungoma, in western Kenya, PATH uses Magnet Theater to help communities prevent HIV transmission. Now HIV and sex—once taboo topics of conversation—have become accepted subjects, laying the groundwork for societal attitudes to change and for new social norms to take hold.

To raise awareness of HIV, AIDS, and related issues, PATH also brought Kenya's top hip-hop musicians together to write and record a song for young people. The song, entitled "Vumilia: Take Control," encourages young people to be proactive in their relationships and to protect themselves against HIV. It promotes abstinence, being faithful, using condoms, and making healthy choices. The song was produced in conjunction with eQuest, a nationwide, mobile phone–based contest for young people aged 15 to 24. Contestants received questions about HIV and AIDS on their mobile phones, looked for the answers in a special eQuest column printed in the newspapers, and then sent in their answers by text message. Questions were focused on HIV prevention, living with HIV, stigma, voluntary counseling and testing, and care and support for individuals living with HIV. The contest was linked to youth role models and personalities in music, sports, politics, and entertainment. Contestants who submitted correct answers had the opportunity to win sought-after prizes.

National Health Policy

Some NGOs have the capacity to advocate for evidence-based changes in a country's standard practice of care. While much of this work entails transferring technical knowledge and skills through training courses, another aspect involves creating a policy climate to accept and actively support the intended changes. Generally, this occurs through policy and guideline changes at the national or, in more decentralized systems, the regional or provincial levels. The case profile below illustrates the complex but ultimately successful path that one NGO took to refine national health policy in South Africa.

Spotlight on South Africa: Cervical Cancer Screening for All

In South Africa, where cervical cancer is the leading cause of cancer-related mortality, the Women's Health Project (WHP) decided to take on the issue of persuading the government to develop and implement a cervical cancer screening policy. The university-based NGO focused on this issue out of concern over unequal access to preventive health services: more affluent women were able to access Pap smears from private providers on a regular basis, whereas less affluent women were not able to access these services in the public sector. In planning this intervention, the WHP identified four groups of key stakeholders: women, health workers, health system managers, and private practitioners and academics. To influence policymakers, they addressed the concerns of each key stakeholder group in a number of ways (table 2).

Table 2. Policy change strategies by key stakeholder group.

Stakeholder group	Strategy used
Women	Developed workshop manual and facilitator training for lay women to raise awareness of cervical cancer prevention with their peers.
Health workers	Developed a participatory workshop method to manage change and build awareness of gender inequality and how to address it at the clinic level.[3,]
Health system managers	Analyzed cost and effectiveness of cervical screening and availability of facilities. Conducted a literature review of impact of cervical screening programs worldwide.
Private practitioners and academics	Built support for an effective and efficient screening strategy of three times per lifetime as opposed to yearly Pap smears through draft policy.

Once the needs of each key stakeholder group had been addressed, WHP took advantage of consultations that were already taking place in the country as part of the 1994 Women's Health Conference, which was run by a coalition of NGOs and managed by the WHP. The process culminated with a policy conference where the policy proposal was finalized and then popularized with press briefings and dissemination of reference materials in local languages.

At this point, the government needed to endorse and agree to implement the policy. This was achieved—in part because some of the key stakeholders who had been involved in the consultative process became part of the newly elected African National Congress (ANC) government during the 1994 elections. In addition, the WHP was part of the ANC's Women's Health Commission and was instrumental in getting the cervical screening strategy into the ANC's health plan.

The government established the National Cancer Control Advisory Committee and made cervical cancer one of its priority areas. The WHP was invited to be a member of this committee. In 1997, the full proposal for a National Cancer Control Strategy encompassing the "three times per lifetime" free screening services for all women aged 30 years or older was presented to the Department of Health. After a period of internal debate, the government accepted the strategy in 1999.

The challenge of how to implement the policy remained, however. To remedy this, the WHP partnered with the Department of Health, the Women's Health Research Unit at the University of Cape Town, and an international NGO, EngenderHealth, to conduct operations research to develop cervical screening processes, protocols, training manuals, and systems. The results of this work are well documented elsewhere [19-21].

Case Study and table adapted from: Klugman:2000.[4]

---

[3] This method was subsequently field-tested by WHO in two multicenter studies in Africa. The manual is Fonn: 1995 [18].

Global Health Policy

NGOs—particularly transnational NGOs—have become key players in setting the priorities around global reproductive health policy. The effect of their participation can be seen in the changes that took place during several key international reproductive health conferences organized by the United Nations in the 1990s, including the International Conference on Population and Development (ICPD) in Cairo in 1994, the Fourth World Conference on Women in Beijing in 1995, and the World Summit for Social Development in Copenhagen in 1995.

The Women's Caucus was held separately during these major conferences and was comprised of women's NGOs from around the world. As a result of excellent and attentive communication between NGO-based women's health advocates and the official country delegations to the meetings, the Women's Caucus made a strong and lasting impact on women's health policy recommendations. After these conferences, global health policy shifted from focusing on population control as the underlying reason to implement reproductive health programs to a paradigm based on reproductive and sexual health and rights. This paradigm recognized the importance of gender equity. For example, the ICPD *Programme of Action* included a variety of forward-thinking areas such as:

- A comprehensive definition of reproductive health, including sexual health, that is integrated with primary health services for all.
- Recognition of adolescents' rights to all reproductive and sexual health services, including sexual education and full protection against unwanted pregnancy and STIs.
- Identification of "Gender Equality, Equity, and Empowerment of Women" as a distinct chapter and valuable end in itself.
- Shared male responsibility for childcare, housework, and reproductive and sexual health.
- A definition of reproductive health services that includes not only family planning but also prenatal and obstetric care, infertility treatment, and prevention and treatment of HIV/AIDS, STIs, and gynecological cancers.
- Recognition that the elimination of all forms of violence against women, including female genital mutilation, is integral to reproductive health.

These new perspectives represented a tremendous shift in the policy environment that prevailed at the time. During the conference, groups that held either fundamentalist or populationist viewpoints hotly contested the emergence of this paradigm. Transnational women's NGOs countered these arguments effectively. At the ICPD, the Women's Environment and Development Organization convened a large, public Women's Caucus outside the meeting while the International Women's Health Coalition mobilized a network of lobbyists and NGO delegates who worked behind the scenes to draft appropriate text [23].

Today, in spite of these major policy advancements, sexual and reproductive health is startlingly absent from the Millennium Development Goals (MDGs) and associated efforts to measure development progress and ensure sustainable and equitable development worldwide

---

[4] Klugman, B. The role of NGOs as agents for change. *Development Dialogue,* 2000 1(2), 95–120.

[24,25]. NGOs are actively working to redress this omission. European NGOs have already formed a transnational NGO for sexual and reproductive health and rights, population, and development to highlight the natural linkages between the MDGs and the goals of the ICPD *Programme of Action* [26]. They have sponsored conferences that bring together a range of participants to examine and assess progress and challenges in ensuring that the central goals of the ICPD are prioritized within the interpretation and implementation of the MDGs.

Resource Mobilization and Allocation

Some NGOs direct their policy and advocacy work with governments to reallocating budgets and resources toward high-priority problems for which there are feasible solutions. NGOs also work with communities to mobilize resources, often by initiating revolving community funds. These types of funds have been used to support health interventions as diverse as urgent transport during obstetrical emergencies to palliative care for women with late-stage cervical cancer.

Microcredit and Related Loans

Some NGOs also establish community-based microcredit financing schemes. Through microcredit financing, very poor families are provided with very small, repayable loans to help them engage in productive activities or grow their small businesses. Over time, these schemes have evolved to offer microfinance options such as credit, savings, and insurance [27].

The use of microcredit to provide "living loans" is an interesting variation on more traditional microcredit financing approaches. For example, Heifer International, an NGO devoted to alleviating hunger and poverty in a sustainable way, uses a modified version of microcredit in all its programs by providing a living loan of livestock. The living loan brings with it the benefits of milk, wool, draft power, eggs, and offspring to pass on to another farmer.

In Nicaragua, Hurricane Mitch destroyed many communities on the banks of the El Zopilote River, forcing everyone to relocate. Several families—which were mostly headed by women—learned how to turn the hen they received into a major source of income. The goal of the project was not only to feed these families but also to provide another, more consistent way for them to make a living. Chickens are effective income-producing animals because, by the time they are six months old, they can lay up to 200 eggs a year, and their manure makes organic fertilizer for vegetable gardens. Initially, training and supplies were provided to the women before a single chicken was distributed. The women learned how to build portable hen houses using local resources and how to feed and care for their hens. The women promised to repay their living loan by donating one or more of their animal's offspring to another family in need [28].

Monitoring Quality of Care and Responsiveness

NGOs can also facilitate communication between health care systems and the clients that they serve. Communication can reflect the realities of the client population as well as their perceptions of the quality of care being offered. Most important, local NGOs that are working with communities on a daily basis can gain an understanding of the sociocultural determinants of women's health and the way that gender equity, in particular, may impact it.

For example, the NGO Conservation of Cutivireni Heritage (ACPC) is dedicated to protecting the natural homelands and maintaining the cultural heritage of the Asháninka people who live in the Peruvian Amazon. With assistance from the International Women's Health Coalition, an international NGO, the ACPC implemented a self-assessment methodology known as "autodiagnósticos" that used games and group exercises to help indigenous women analyze their lives, identify their health needs, reflect on the health care they receive, and give feedback to the health care system. As a result, ACPC is now coordinating a concerted effort between the community and the local health system to address the cultural, linguistic, and gender gaps that prevent Asháninka women from realizing their right to sexual and reproductive health. The Association is collaborating with local women on community-level projects and advocacy efforts to address women's health needs, training local women who speak Asháninka and Spanish to serve as community health promoters, and leading efforts to ensure that local health providers—who are primarily Spanish-speaking men—approach their work with cultural and gender sensitivity [29].

ENVISIONING THE FUTURE ROLE OF NGOS

When it comes to women's health, an NGO may focus on only one or on several of the areas described above. Given how closely NGOs work with government partners, many important questions arise as to what their role should be:

- To what extent should NGOs undertake the role of government to provide health services?
- To what extent should they refrain from direct service delivery and instead advocate for increased effort by governments in this sector?
- Whose responsibility is it to provide a functioning health system that makes services available and accessible to the majority of the population?
- Whose responsibility is it to make policymakers and program planners aware of the health care needs and solutions of overlooked populations and support them in making rational, evidence-based decisions?

These are among the most fundamental questions raised in discussions about the involvement of NGOs in international development and the health sector.

NGOs may be constrained by both internal and external factors in their potential to address women's health issues. Internal factors may include changing technical and institutional capacity that affects organizational growth and development, internal politics, lack of autonomy, and financial instability. External factors may include changing policies and priorities, shifting donor priorities, inability to scale up promising approaches, limitations common to low-resource settings, changing global economy, and the extent to which NGO activities are formally recognized and integrated into public health systems. The theoretical debates about NGOs often revolve around one or more of these factors.

KEY CHALLENGES

Organizational Growth and Development

NGOs, like other organizations, wrestle with concerns regarding organizational growth and development. One study conducted in Bangladesh investigated how NGOs make strategic decisions on the location of service delivery sites [30]. The conclusion was that NGOs in Bangladesh typically establish new programs where they had no programs previously. The choice of site was usually not affected by whether another NGO was already present and offering the same services. The study showed that, in general, NGOs initiated services in areas that provided a new location for their own organization and these decisions were not always consistent with other factors such as local needs or overall service provision rates.

This illustrates the complex nature of NGO decision-making when targeting an urgent health need while navigating practical realities such as the desire to work in environments where the NGO can have impact, where there is absorptive capacity, or where the policy environment will facilitate successful programming.

Assessing and Strengthening Performance

NGOs must be responsive to differing levels of data and evaluation needs. They must demonstrate programmatic effectiveness while retaining legitimacy in the view of both their intended beneficiary and key stakeholders. Increasingly NGOs are required to use a sophisticated blend of evaluation techniques to assess their overall performance against predetermined input, output, outcome, and impact benchmarks. Most donors have requirements that NGOs must demonstrate managerial, financial, and bureaucratic accountability and transparency.

Driven by the increasingly competitive donor and political environment in which scrutiny is applied to financial systems, program results, and accreditation, NGOs are becoming increasingly professionalized and more attentive to demonstrating the impact of their initiatives through project design, outcome measurement, program monitoring, and evaluation. Local NGOs address this situation by retaining qualified technical personnel, often locally trained, who work with external sources of funding to address specific issues in a measurable way. National or international NGOs often partner with local NGOs to execute activities on the ground.

For example in Bihar, India, 19 local NGOs were selected to work with Pathfinder International to improve the health and welfare of young mothers and their children by changing traditional customs of early childbearing. This three-year project was implemented in 452 villages and reached more than 90,000 young people and 100,000 parents and other community adults with messages about delaying and spacing the birth of their children. During the course of the project, Pathfinder provided orientation and training in reproductive health and family planning as well as project management, monitoring, and administration to build NGO capacity to the level needed to implement such a demanding project [31]. In return, the smaller NGOs were critically important in implementing the project.

When national, regional, or local NGOs attempt to respond to donor requirements in a rigorous way, they may face internal conflict from members or staff who believe that the organization is losing its connection to an issue or a population that they are serving. The criticism is often that the resources spent measuring, monitoring, and evaluating the work diminish the organization's ability to address the needs of target groups. This viewpoint is fostered by the high level of attention and resources required to meet the needs of large donors who require unique, very specific frameworks for monitoring and evaluation efforts, often without adequate funding and minimal coordination. One study of Dutch, Bolivian, and Peruvian NGOs posited that the need to assess NGO performance in terms of impact paradoxically may be a root cause of NGO inability to remain true to their intended mission [32].

Additional reflection suggests that when the overriding mission is to reduce poverty, for example, community need may not be the primary consideration; the political economy of aid and development, religious and political geography, the transnational networks in which these institutions are embedded, and the social networks and life experiences of NGO professionals must also be considered [33]. Thus, a question arises: when are NGOs the best vehicles to meet the needs of the underserved?

Sustainability

There is little doubt that NGOs contribute to improving the general health and welfare of society. The potential for these activities to be sustained over the long term is often questioned, however. Almost all major donor agencies now require that sustainability plans be developed during project design.

International NGOs can approach the issue of sustainability in a variety of ways. Some projects are structured at the outset to revert wholly to government ownership. While this approach may sound appealing, it may be difficult to achieve. Sustainability has been accomplished if an NGO's activities are structured so that their financial contributions gradually diminish over time and are covered by increasing government commitments. To ensure sustainability of services, the costs of the project are gradually transferred from the NGO to the government on a yearly percentage basis. For example, during the first year of the project, 20 percent of all project costs might be borne by the government; by the end of the project, the government would bear 100 percent of the costs associated with implementing and monitoring the service.

It is critical to note that, at some level, the question of program sustainability becomes irrelevant. As noted by the United Nations, it is not realistic to expect NGOs to support themselves and their programs without external funding assistance. The UN specifically states that as "long as there are unserved, underserved, marginalized, poorer persons who are unable to obtain the basic necessities of life in many developing nations, external assistance will be needed. This assistance must reach poorer persons—through those institutions, governments

or NGOs, which are working in the field to provide quality reproductive health services [37]."
This focus is more appropriate when looking for ways to ensure that the change, intervention,
or service is sustainable, rather than the NGO itself. By its very nature, a funded entity is not
sustainable unless its funding source is. This is as true for governments as it is for private
companies and NGOs..

Representation and Accountability

An overriding set of issues for local and national NGOs (or coalitions of NGOs) pertains
to representation and accountability in the local context. A related issue is the ability to
influence existing health policy. For instance, can a local NGO, created and staffed by
members of the local elite, really represent and advocate for disenfranchised or marginalized
populations and influence the policy process? The Centre for African Studies and the Task
Force on NGO Partnerships undertook a study to explore reproductive health NGO
leadership, classification, and management structure in a representative sample of 11
countries in sub-Saharan Africa. Results suggest that most African NGOs rely too heavily on
the vision and commitment of their founding members, are reticent to embrace the
organizational skills of possibly better-educated younger leaders, and have limited
accountability to end beneficiaries as well as donors [40].

These issues of representation and accountability are perhaps exacerbated by the
increasing need for NGOs to professionalize their approach and to add expertise to their
organization. Improving technical capacity and the ability to monitor and evaluate
programmatic and policy efforts requires specific skill sets. Individuals learn the appropriate
skills in institutions of higher learning, either in the country or abroad. Individuals who obtain
such educations generally come from more privileged backgrounds.

Critical debate around the ability of NGO workers to accurately reflect the voices of
poor, minority, and rural people has emerged. Doubt also has been expressed about whether
the NGO structure is conducive to allowing disadvantaged people to participate more fully in
any discussion of their livelihoods and future, particularly as part of NGO rural development
efforts [41,42]. Positive trends have been observed for NGOs actively reaching out to
underserved communities where people live in remote areas, informal and squatter
settlements, and poor communities [15]. Many more local NGOs are embracing rights-based
and social justice values as avenues to work with these types of marginalized populations. As
these NGOs become more successful in "growing" their internal leadership, the ability of the
leaders to accurately reflect the voice of marginalized populations becomes a real concern.
NGOs will need to respond to this reality and seek creative ways to maintain their
representative voice.

Politicized Foreign Assistance

The politicization of foreign assistance is not a new phenomenon. For many years, the
biggest bilateral recipients of all direct US foreign assistance have been Israel and Egypt for
so-called "development" efforts. At the time of writing, the inclusion of militaristic thinking
relative to foreign assistance has become more apparent. The decision made in 2006 by the

United States Secretary of State, Condoleeza Rice, to align US foreign assistance with security needs is an instructive example. Dr. Rice stated that "Our foreign assistance must help people get results. The resources we commit must empower developing countries to strengthen security, to consolidate democracy, to increase trade and investment, and to improve the lives of their people [48]."

The effect of this realignment on the work being undertaken by NGOs in the health sector is unknown. One can surmise, however, that as more assistance dollars go toward democratization and free market efforts, fewer dollars will be available for delivery of health interventions. Likewise, in such a political climate, new foreign assistance funding may carry a more strictly defined purpose that aligns closely with the current political agenda. In this setting, non-aligned countries may find it more difficult to attract foreign aid from countries such as the United States.

Religious Fundamentalism

In some parts of the world, religious fundamentalism is also becoming a global force that needs to be better understood. Writing in *New Scientist*, MacKenzie commented that "pluralism and tolerance of other faiths, non-traditional gender roles and sexual behavior, reliance on human reason rather than divine revelation, and democracy, which grants power to people rather than God [49]." In this context, fundamentalist views may define the content, approach, and, ultimately, the existence of women's health initiatives in many settings. When fundamentalism leads to a division of genders, women's rights and women's health in particular, suffer. Some people, who may have key religious and societal positions, may also believe that science is contrary to religion, and this compounds the difficulties that NGOs face when delivering evidence-based health programs. It is an issue, for example, in the current debate over condom use and abstinence in stemming the AIDS epidemic [50]. As these views are integrated into governmental policy, NGOs will need to become more adept at navigating the resultant sea changes that are bound to occur.

Human Rights

A human rights perspective demanding increased gender equity has been nominally integrated into women's health initiatives since the 1990s. Nonetheless, many of the core gender-based issues pertinent to women's health remain unresolved. For instance, WHO recently conducted the *Multi-country Study on Women's Health and Domestic Violence against Women*, which was carried out with 24,000 women in 10 countries. The study results confirm that women around the world are at significant risk of physical and sexual violence, that much of this violence is hidden, and that it causes serious—often long-term—health consequences. Women who reported violence were more likely to report poor general health and more physical symptoms of ill health, emotional distress, miscarriages, and abortions. They also were more likely to have considered or attempted suicide. In 13 of the 15 study sites, one-third to three-quarters of women had been physically or sexually assaulted by an intimate partner. At some sites, as many as 28 percent of women who had been pregnant had been assaulted during pregnancy [51]. Clearly, these underlying factors must be addressed by NGOs for broader health inequities to be overcome.

KEY OPPORTUNITIES

Collaboration with the Private Sector

More and more, donors are encouraging NGOs to reach out to private-sector partners as a way to provide project sustainability. This requires NGOs to change the way they often view themselves. They must become more entrepreneurial and seek opportunities to provide their services, as well as meet the needs of their service consumers.

Although this approach may be appealing at a theoretical level, many NGOs working in women's health have little capacity to engage with the private sector. One study of the 16 largest reproductive health NGOs in Uganda found that most of them had low skill or capacity for strategic planning, marketing, human resource management, and governance, and they had limited funding options. All of these characteristics are necessary capacities if NGOs are to successfully negotiate sustainable arrangements with private-sector partners [34]. Likewise, an assessment of 35 NGOs involved in the corporate-sponsored "Smiling Sun" community health clinic system in Bangladesh identified weaknesses in institutional sustainability, particularly in self-government and management practices [35].

Collaboration with the Community

Ensuring the sustainability of community-based programs implemented unilaterally by local NGOs may be even less straightforward. Sometimes the community-based program can be sustained over the long term while the local NGO cannot. One way to achieve sustainability of both the community-based programs and the local NGOs that implement them is to build the capacity of the NGOs so they can respond to changing community needs in a flexible manner. Another way to ensure program sustainability is to build the capacity of the community to allow eventual handover of ownership and ongoing management of the program, thereby allowing the NGO to withdraw [36].

Collaboration with Government

The majority of countries in low-resource settings encourage active collaboration with NGOs, particularly international NGOs that have a relatively large resource base. In some cases, NGOs fulfill large parts of the government's role of providing adequate health services and disease surveillance. This is particularly common in countries where services are limited due to recent armed conflict or lack of adequate funding to reach all underserved areas.

At the time of this writing, Cambodia presents an interesting case study. The government is attempting to work with NGOs in a novel way so that high-quality government health services become more available and accessible to the population. The country is still recovering from the effects of the Khmer Rouge, the resulting destruction of hospitals, and a severe lack of medical professionals. To counter this, international donors currently provide about two-thirds of the public health–sector spending and have constructed abundant hospitals and clinics. The services remain underutilized, however. In 1999, the Cambodian Ministry of Health began to think differently about how to work with the international NGO community. The ministry decided to contract services to five NGOs and to allow them to run parts of the health system. The NGOs are paid based on their performance in improving services. Last year, the government began transferring the ministry's budget directly from the national treasury to the NGO contractors to restrict corrupt practices. The NGOs are using incentives such as paying for provider punctuality and for reaching immunization targets, and they are complementing staff salaries with revenues gained through provider fees. Initial feedback suggests that this approach may be successful in creating a health system that provides good-quality services to satisfied clients.[5]

Reconfiguring Reliance on International Aid

At one time or another, many countries have chosen to openly acknowledge their desire to avoid dependence on international aid, often for political reasons. When this happens, international aid that addresses specific needs that cannot be met internally may be no longer be welcomed. In some notable cases, such as in Eritrea in 2005, aid was designed to minimize continued external support, and aid that complemented and strengthened—instead of replaced—the country's institutional capacity to implement projects was preferred. The Eritrean government also insisted on retaining ownership of all projects so that they and the benefits they achieved would be sustainable and not subject to unpredictable shifts in donor priorities or financial commitments. This meant that, theoretically, the government of Eritrea, rather than NGOs, took the lead in identifying problems, setting priorities, and designing solutions for them [39]. This example is indicative of a growing trend for national governments resolve to become self-sustaining.

"Cutting-Edge" NGOs in Action

NGOs that wish to effectively and efficiently address women's health must embrace a comprehensive programming approach in their work. The most effective NGOs will maximize the impact of each dollar spent on health; use appropriate, evidence-based, and sustainable interventions; advocate for policy change, and partner with local groups to implement a collaborative approach to address a specific issue. Based on its many years of experience, PATH has developed core principles to guide its development efforts towards successful outcomes. These principles for obtaining effective health solutions in low-resource settings include developing solutions that have a measurable impact on health and are scientifically and technologically sound, locally sustainable, culturally relevant, and gender equitable [47].

---

[5] Dugger, C. Cambodia tries nonprofit path to health care. *New York Times*. January 8, 2006.

The recognition that NGOs can improve their effectiveness by fostering public-private partnerships is an area of increasing interest. In this regard, the challenge and opportunity for NGOs working at the cutting edge is to identify strategies for effectively linking with multiple players across sectors to accelerate the introduction of health interventions. In response, public-private partnerships—in which pharmaceutical companies, biotech firms, manufacturers, and other companies partner with NGOs, academic institutions, and international agencies to conduct research and develop drugs and/or vaccines—have become more widespread [43]. At the time of this writing, there are nearly 100 of these public-private partnerships devoted solely to drug development for the purposes of improving global health, particularly with respect to treating neglected diseases—such as malaria, tuberculosis, dengue fever, and schistosomiasis—that are prevalent in low-resource settings [44].

PATH is an example of an international NGO that works in a range of countries with local communities, regional and national governments, the broader donor and policymaker community, and private industry partners. Together, these groups work to understand health issues and develop, test, and advocate for appropriate solutions, particularly health technologies for low-resource settings. With its well-established emphasis on developing pubic-private partnerships, PATH serves as an important model for this new trend. For example, PATH is taking the lead on working with industry partners in an integrated effort to accelerate the development and introduction of new tests and vaccines for the human papillomavirus (HPV) to screen and immunize women against cervical cancer. Working with private-sector collaborators, PATH is committed to making rapid, accurate, and affordable HPV tests accessible in low-resource settings as an alternative to Pap smear screening, which requires complex and expensive infrastructure [45]. Partnerships between PATH and pharmaceutical manufacturers are being developed to facilitate early introduction of an HPV vaccine in selected developing countries, develop a case for investing in an HPV vaccine, address country- and region-specific programmatic issues, and address information needs.

The involvement of NGOs in drug and vaccine development through public-private partnerships is just one aspect of the increasing complexity of the global health field. NGOs that are involved in public-private partnerships must also contend with previously unforeseen issues such as the ethics of clinical trials and medical research and the ever-changing nature of the biotechnology field. How do NGOs continue to play their traditional role in this environment, and what new roles are emerging? In an effort to address these issues, PATH developed guiding principles on collaboration with the private sector that outline tangible methods for achieving the maximum sustainable benefit for public health in low-resource settings. The principles are based on engaging private-sector collaborators to apply their development, manufacturing, and distribution strengths toward innovative technologies that would not otherwise be their priority [46].

Spotlight on the ACCP: Comprehensive Programming for Women's Health

Until recently, cervical cancer prevention has been a neglected aspect of women's health in low-resource settings—primarily because of the high cost related to screening with Pap smears. Yet cervical cancer kills more than 288,000 women each year and disproportionately affects the poorest, most vulnerable women. At least 80 percent of cervical cancer deaths occur in developing countries, with most occurring in the poorest regions—South Asia, sub-

Saharan Africa, and parts of Latin America. Several international NGOs identified the possibility of addressing this issue by providing an evidence base for the use of alternative screening techniques that were less expensive than standard methods.

Beginning in 1999 with funding from the Bill and Melinda Gates Foundation, five international organizations—PATH, EngenderHealth, the International Agency for Research on Cancer (IARC), JHPIEGO, and the Pan American Health Organization (PAHO)—have implemented the Alliance for Cervical Cancer Prevention (ACCP). With a shared goal of preventing cervical cancer in developing countries, the ACCP project worked at all levels of the health system.

Each of the five partners led at least one large research or demonstration project for a cervical cancer prevention program. With assistance from local NGO partners, formative research on what women and health care providers know, believe, and do was the starting point for designing more effective cervical cancer programs for each country setting. Surveys, focus group discussions, interviews, and other techniques were employed to ensure that programs reflected community perspectives and needs. These projects demonstrated strategies for community involvement, alternatives to Pap smears for screening, affordable treatment methods, and advocacy materials. Each project was based on a solid platform of design, measurement, and evaluation that allowed comparison of results across countries.

At the international level, the ACCP has developed advocacy materials as the results of the demonstration projects emerged and raised awareness about cervical cancer worldwide. The ACCP organizations produced joint publications and materials such as fact sheets and PowerPoint presentations that could be used by health advocates, as well as scientific publications in peer-reviewed journals that reached international opinion leaders in the fields of gynecology, oncology, and public health. Eventually, influential international bodies such as the WHO, IARC, PAHO, the National Cancer Institute, and the Federation of Gynecology and Obstetrics lent their support by inviting presentations and joint publications.

Local support for cervical cancer prevention and learning how best to integrate programs into wider national health care systems also are key priority areas. For example, in several countries, ACCP partners, acting collaboratively with local groups, established planning and advisory groups to assist with cervical cancer prevention projects, explore revisions to national policies, and seek increased financial support for cervical cancer prevention.

Local NGOs were able to catalyze projects in their local areas through ACCP's Small Grants Program, which provided funding for 42 small projects from 1999 through 2004. In most cases, funding was used to develop awareness about cervical cancer or to provide an opportunity to pilot screening and treatment services. For example, the *African Organization for Reproductive Health and Social Development* implemented a pilot project initiating a cervical cancer screening program in Kordofan state, Sudan, using a screening technique called visual inspection with acetic acid (VIA) and cryotherapy for treating precancerous lesions. The organization anticipates that the results of the project will influence policies and guidelines on cancer prevention and encourage the reallocation of resources to implement these services in a national screening program.

In implementing a comprehensive programming approach to cervical cancer prevention through education, screening, treatment, and advocacy, the NGOs in the ACCP have demonstrated an ability to work successfully in the current environment. For more information about the ACCP, visit *www.alliance-cxca.org.*

CONCLUSION

NGOs have proven themselves to be key players in the provision of women's health. They have expanded access and use of key women's health interventions, and they provide a voice for marginalized populations, many of whom are women. They also broker effective partnerships with private- and public-sector entities and lead new joint ventures in addressing some of the world's most serious chronic and complex health issues.

Fortunately, the NGO voice is becoming more powerful. The increasing participation of international NGO leaders in global economic and financial gatherings and in the leadership of global coalitions addressing key health issues demonstrates the contributions that NGOs can make. A clear and important leadership role for NGOs in setting a global agenda for the creation of a healthy future for women is emerging, and the potential for a leadership role in finding solutions to women's health problems has never been greater.

ACRONYMS

ACCP	Alliance for Cervical Cancer Prevention
ACPC	Conservation of Cutivireni Heritage
CBO	Community Based Organization
CSO	Civil Society Organization
HPV	human papillomavirus
IARC	International Agency for Research on Cancer
ICPD	International Conference on Population and Development
IPPF	International Planned Parenthood Federation
JHPIEGO	
MDG	Millennium Development Goals
NGOs	Non-governmental Organization
PAHO	Pan American Health Organization
PATH	Program for Appropriate Technology in Health
PVO	Private Voluntary Organization
WASN	Women and AIDS Support Network
WHO	World Health Organization

SUGGESTED READING LIST

Hartmann, B. *Reproductive Rights and Wrongs*. Boston, MA: South End Press; 1995.

Hancock, G. *Lords of Poverty: The Power, Prestige, and Corruption of the International Aid Business*. London, UK: MacMillan London Limited; 1989.

Anderson, M. *Do No Harm: How Aid Can Support Peace—or War.* Boulder, CO: Lynn Rienner Pub; 1999.

Edwards, M; Hulme, D eds. *Non-Governmental Organisations—Accountability and Performance: Beyond the Magic Bullet*. London, UK: Earthscan; 1995.

Hulme, D; Edwards, M eds. *Too close for comfort? NGOs, Donors and the State.* Oxford, UK: MacMillan 1997.

Fowler, A ed. Questioning Partnership: the reality of AID and NGO relations. *IDS Bulletin,* 2000 31(3).

Edwards, M; Hulme, D eds. *Making a difference: NGOs and development in a changing world.* London, UK: Earthscan; 1992.

Chambers, R. *NGOs and Development: The Primacy of the Personal.* Brighton, UK: University of Sussex; 1995. IDS Working Paper 14.

REFERENCES

[1]   Directory of Development Organizations website. Available at: *www.devdir.org.* Accessed on February 22, 2006.

[2]   Idealist.org website. Available at *www.idealist.org.* Accessed on February 22, 2006.

[3]   United Nations Development Program (UNDP). Deepening democracy at the global level. In: UNDP. *Human Development Report 2002: Deepening Democracy in a Fragmenting World.* Oxford, UK: Oxford University Press; 2002.

[4]   Gellert, G. Non-governmental organizations in international health: past successes, future challenges. *International Journal of Health Planning and Management,* 1996 11(1), 1931.

[5]   Willetts, P. *What is a non-governmental organization?* In UNESCO CSI/2001/DP1. Geneva: WHO; 2001.

[6]   Categorizing NGOs page. NGO Research Guide website. Available at: *http://docs.lib.duke.edu/igo/guides/ngo/define.htm.* Accessed January 9 2006.

[7]   World Health Organization (WHO). *WHO and Civil Society: Linking for Better Health.* WHO/CSI/2002/DP1. Geneva: WHO; 2002.

[8]   WHO. *Understanding Civil Society Issues for WHO, Civil Society Initiative.* CSI/2002/DP2. Geneva: WHO; 2002.

[9]   WHO. *Strategic Alliances: The Role of Civil Society in Health.* CSI/2001/DP1. Geneva: WHO; 2001.

[10]   Walls, D. *Acting Globally: Transnational NGOs and Political Networks.* Albuquerque: Southwest Research and Information Center; 1998. The Workbook Fall/Winter.

[11]   Harcourt, W ed. Globalization, Reproductive Health and Rights. *Development,*2003 46(2).

[12]   Launching the Legacy: 300,000 and Counting: Are Transnational NGOs Changing the World page. Moynihan Institute of Global Affairs website. Available at: *www.maxwell.syr.edu/moynihan/symposiaQ2.html.* Accessed January 24, 2006.

[13]   Cossey, M. Tsunami aid maroons Thai sex workers. *Women's e News.* January, 8, 2006. Available at: http://*www.womensenews.org/article.cfm/dyn/aid/2592/contex t/archive. Accessed on: February 22, 2006.*

[14]   The Female Condom in Zimbabwe: The Interplay of Research, Advocacy, and Government Action page. Population Council website. Available at: *http://www.popcouncil.org/horizons/ressum/fczimbresadvgovt/index.html.* Accessed February 22, 2006.

[15] Annotated Bibliography on Civil Society and Health page. Training and Research Support Centre website. Available at: *http://www.tarsc.org/WHOCSI/index.php.* Accessed February 22, 2006.

[16] International Planned Parenthood website. Available at: *www.ippf.org.* Accessed February 22, 2006.

[17] Family Planning page. Population Services International website. Available at: *http://www.psi.org/our_programs/family_planning.html.* Accessed January 24, 2006.

[18] Fonn, S; Xaba, M. *Health Workers for Change: A Manual to Improve Quality of Care.* Geneva: WHO; 1995.

[19] EngenderHealth. *Cervical Health Implementation Project, South Africa. Technical Report.* Cape Town: University of the Witwatersrand, University of Cape Town, and EngenderHealth; 2003.

[20] CHIP. *Implementing Cervical Screening in South Africa, Volume I: A Guide for Programme Managers.* South Africa: EngenderHealth; 2004.

[21] Cervical Health Implementation Project (CHIP). *Implementing Cervical Screening in South Africa, Volume II: A Guide for Trainers.* South Africa: EngenderHealth; 2004.

[22] Klugman, B. The role of NGOs as agents for change. *Development Dialogue,* 2000 1(2), 95–120.

[23] Petchesky, R. *Reproductive and sexual Rights: Charting the Course of Transnational Women's NGOs.* Geneva: UNRISD; 2000.

[24] Crossette, B. *Reproductive Health and the Millennium Development Goals: The Missing Link.* Menlo Park, CA: Hewlett Foundation; 2004. Available at: *http://www.hewlett.org/Programs/Population/Publications/crossettereport.htm.*

[25] Sexuality Information and Education Council of the United States (SIECUS). *The Underlying Millennium Development Goal: Universal Access to Reproductive Health Services.* New York: SIECUS; 2005. Making the Connection—News and Views on Sexuality: Education, Health, and Rights, Volume 4, Issue 1.

[26] The European NGOs for Sexual and Reproductive Health and Rights, Population, and Development website. Available at: *www.eurongos.org.* Accessed February 22, 2006.

[27] The Microfinance Gateway website. Available at: *www.microfinancegateway.org.* Accessed February 22, 2006.

[28] "Today I am the Breadwinner" page. Heifer International website. Available at: *http://www.heifer.org/site/c.edJRKQNiFiG/b.201441/.* Accessed February 22, 2006.

[29] Mogollón, G; Haver, A. *Sexual and Reproductive Rights and Health: Perceptions, Problems, and Priorities Identified by Asháninka Women of Peru's Rio Ene Region.* New York: International Women's Health Coalition; 2003. Available at: *www.iwhc.org/resources/acpc2003feature.cfm.*

[30] Fruttero, A; Gauri, V. The strategic choices of NGOs: location decision in rural Bangladesh. *Journal of Development Studies.* 2005 41(5), 759–787.

[31] Wilder, J; Masilamani, R; Daniel, E. *Promoting Change in the Reproductive Behaviour of Youth: Pathfinder International's PRACHAR Project, Bihar, India.* Watertown, MA: Pathfinder International; 2005. Available at: *http://www.pathfind.org/site/Doc Server/India-Prachar_Project.pdf?docID=4261.*

[32] Bebbington, A. Donor-NGO relations and representations of livelihood in nongovernmental aid chains. *World Development,* 2005 33(6), 937–950.

[33] Bebbington, A. NGOs and uneven development: geographies of development intervention. *Progress in Human Geography,* 2004 28(6), 725–745.

[34] Mugisha, F; Birungi, H; Askew, I. Are reproductive health NGOs in Uganda able to engage in the health SWAp? *International Journal of Health Planning and Management,* 2005 20, 227–238.

[35] NGO Service Delivery Program (NSDP). *Scoring NGO Development and Tailoring TA.* Watertown, MA: NSDP; 2006. NSDP Brief #3.

[36] Kahn, A; Hare, L. *Sustaining the Benefits: A Field Guide for Sustaining Reproductive and Child Health Services.* Washington, DC: CEDPA; 2003.

[37] United Nations Population Fund (UNFPA). Report on the roundtable on partnership with civil society to implement the ICPD—Programme of Action. Round Table Meeting Dhaka, Bangladesh, 27-30 July 1998. New York: UNFPA; 1998.

[38] Dugger, C. Cambodia tries nonprofit path to health care. *New York Times.* January 8, 2006.

[39] NGOs and Aid in Eritrea: A Fact Sheet page. Eritrean Development Foundation website. Available at: *www.edfonline.org/NGO.htm.* Accessed February 22, 2006.

[40] Center for African Family Studies (CAFS). *A Situation Analysis of NGO Governance and Leadership in Eastern, Southern, Central and Western Africa.* Nairobi: CAFS; 2001. Available at: *http://www.cafs.org/sarep.pdf.*

[41] Arellana-Lopez, S; Petras, J. Nongovernmental organizations and poverty alleviation in Boliva. *Development and Change,* 1994 25, 555–568.

[42] Breton, V. The contradictions of rural development NGOS. The trajectory of FEPP in Chimborazo. In: North, L; Cameron, J eds. *Rural Progress, Rural Decay: Neoliberal Adjustment Policies and Local Initiatives.* Bloomfield, Ct: Kumarian Press; 2003; 143–163.

[43] Rockefeller Foundation. *Partnering to Develop New Products for Diseases of Poverty: One Donor's Perspective.* New York: Rockefeller Foundation; 2004. Available at: *http://www.rockfound.org/Library/Partnering_to_Develop_New_Products_for_Disease s_of_Poverty.pdf.*

[44] Cohen, J. The new world of global health. *Science,* 2006 Jan 13 311(5758), 162–167.

[45] Start Project: From the Lab to the Village, Developing Biochemical Tests for Cervical Cancer page. PATH website. Available at: *http://www.path.org/projects/start_ project.php.* Accessed on February 22, 2006.

[46] PATH. *PATH's Guiding Principles for Private-Sector Collaboration.* Seattle: PATH; 2005. Available at: *http://www.path.org/files/ER_gp_collab.pdf.*

[47] PATH. *PATH's Guiding Principles for Achieving Programmatic Impact.* Seattle: PATH; 2005. Available at: *http://www.path.org/files/ER_gp_impact.pdf.*

[48] Fact Sheet: New Direction for U.S. Foreign Assistance [press release]. Washington, DC: USAID; January 19, 2006. Available at: *http://www.usaid.gov/press/factsheets /2006/fs060119.html.*

[49] MacKenzie, D. End of the enlightenment. *New Scientist,* October 8, 2005, 40–43.

[50] Sinding, S. Does CNN (condoms, needles and negotiation) work better than ABC (abstinence, being faithful and condom use) in attacking the AIDS epidemic? *International Family Planning Perspectives,* 2005 31(1), 38–40.

[51] Garcia-Moreno, C; Heise, L; Jansen, HA; Ellsberg, M; Watts, C. Violence against women. *Science,* 2005 Nov 25 310(5752), 1282–1283.

In: Women's Health in the Majority World: Issues and Initiatives   ISBN1-1-60021-493-2
Eds: L. Elit and J. Chamberlain Froese, pp. 179-190   © 2007 Nova Science Publishers, Inc.

Chapter 10

GOVERNMENTS IN HIGH RESOURCE SETTINGS AND INTERNATIONAL WOMEN'S HEALTH

Stephen Lewis[1]

Special envoy from the United Nations for HIV/AIDs in Africa
Social Science Scholar in Residence at McMaster University, Hamilton, Canada

STEPHEN LEWIS' ADDRESS SEPTEMBER 24, 2004 AT THE INTERNATIONAL WOMEN'S AND CHILDRENS' HEALTH CONFERENCE (IWCH) AT THE ROYAL BOTANICAL GARDENS, BURLINGTON, ONTARIO.

IWCH IS SPONSORED BY THE DEPARTMENT OF OBSTETRICS AND GYNECOLOGY AND THE DEGROOTE SCHOOL OF MEDICINE AT MCMASTER UNIVERSITY, AND SISTERS OF ST. JOSEPH HEALTH CARE CENTRE, HAMILTON, ONTARIO, CANADA.

Normally I would engage in that Pavlovian banter to which speakers are addicted at the outset of remarks but I want to use every kernel of the opportunity I have today to address a number of issues, because I can't imagine any theme more compelling than international women's and children's health. When I thought about providing a context for the subject matter, it occurred to me that the millennium development goals were probably the useful centerpiece around which remarks could be constructed. Most of you will know that at the so called millennium general assembly in the year 2000 at the United Nations, the nations around the world came together and through consensus established a series of goals for the year 2015 which spoke primarily to the social and economic imperatives internationally. The goals, while predictable, were uniformly and quite passionately embraced by all of the countries present. They set out to cut poverty in half by the year 2015. Dramatically to reduce infant mortality rates. Dramatically to reduce maternal mortality rates. There's a tremendous effort underway to get girls into school in particular. There was a strong affirmation of the need to achieve gender equality. There was of course a goal to role back the pandemic of HIV and AIDS. There was a seventh goal on environmental preservation. It all came together in the eighth target for 2015, which was to delineate a form of international development cooperation, which would win from the developed world the kind of commitment to the needs of the developing world to overcome so much of the difficulties of the past.

I thought what I would like to do (if you will bear with me) is to deal with each of those omnibus goals, one by one and where appropriate interweave the clear themes of this conference, although it is my own view, that they are indelibly interlinked: Women's Health, Children's Health and the Millennium Development goals.

1. THE GOAL OF CUTTING POVERTY IN HALF BY THE YEAR 2015

It's important to recognize and never to forget, that 1 billion 300 million people on this planet are still living on less than $1 dollar a day. That 3 billion people are living on less than $750 dollars a year. That the impoverishment in many countries and many societies particularly those countries as we describe as developing and least developed countries, the impoverishment is almost unimaginable. That poverty has been intensifying within and between and among countries, rather than diminishing in a universal way across the globe. I think it's important to point out that poverty has indeed has been reduced in a significant fashion in China and South East Asia. But in the more vulnerable parts of the planet, namely sub Saharan Africa, parts of Latin America and many parts of the emerging transitional economies of central and eastern Europe, poverty continues to ransack the future of societies. It is only in Southeast Asia that we have had these major advances. It does seem to me that there are three main policies in response to the epidemic of poverty across the world, which have to be implemented. As I discuss some of these policies and positions during the course of these remarks, I of course want to tie Canada in directly because if I understand it properly, this morning you had a sense of what individuals can do (I think) through Vic Neufeld, you had a sense of what institutions can do from David Zakus, and I want to suggest what Canada might do in the process of dealing with the Millennium Development goals.

1.   If we are to eradicate the worst excrescences of poverty, then the *extraordinary debt burdens*, which the developing countries continue to hold, have to be removed. In other words, you simply have to cancel the debts at they now exist, particularly for the least developed countries which were accrued over a long period of time which they have paid back ten fold through the interest on the debts interminably and which are now held in significant measure by the international financial institutions of the World Bank and international monetary fund, as well as by some major bilateral donors. What is required is a principal voice, the kind of voice, which every Canadian likes to believe, we have. The kind of voice to which Paul Martin attempted to give expression to the nations earlier this week. It needs a voice on a principal stand of removing the debts. If we can eliminate the debt particularly for the countries under siege from communicable diseases, then it means that the money they would spend on the interest on the loans and some of the capital repayment can be plowed back into the social sectors. These countries

---

[1] Contact: Christina Magill, Executive Assistant to Stephen Lewis Email: clmagill@shaw.ca

are so desperate, they don't even mind the relief of the debt being attached to the condition that the money thus saved would go into social priorities.

2.   We to have to do something about the *international trading regimen* because you cannot bring societies a sense of economic growth and stability. When you have an international trading regimen that is so extraordinarily unfair and prejudices the possibilities for growth for all of these societies that are so desperately struggling for growth and survival. The area of world trade which is most offensive and abhorrent is of coarse the agricultural subsidies which are given by the European Union and by the United States of America. $350 billion dollars worth of agricultural subsides every year to maintain the standards and status of western farmers at the expense of African farmers, Latin American farmers, Central American farmers being able to produce and export their agricultural goods. $350 billion dollars is almost seven times what the world gives annually to foreign aid, to official development assistance. One of the ways of characterizing it, sufficiently vivid to remain in one's mind, is to note that every single cow in the European Union is subsidized at a level of $2.00/day. The great majority of Africans live on less than $1/day. If you want to see palpable inequity, that always seemed to me to be a reasonable juxtaposition.

3.   That *objective target for foreign aid of official foreign assistance*, which so many countries said they would adhere to, has somehow to be reached. There are interesting antecedents for Canada. The target which was 0.7, a very famous 0.7, 7/10th of 1% of gross national product, 0.7% of gross national product, that target was actually agreed upon at an International Conference of Industrial Countries chaired by Canada's Lester Pearson in 1969. It is worth noting that from that day to this, 35 years later, only 4 countries with any regularity in this world, have achieved the target: Norway, Denmark, Sweden and Holland. I very much want to believe in reincarnation, because I have enjoyed this life immensely. I would like to come back. If I come back I would like to come back as a Nordic because the Nordics seem to me to be the most extraordinarily equiable and socially aware group of countries in the world. They have all been about the 0.7. Canada has rarely even approximated 0.7; we once got close to 0.5. Now, in the most recent Canadian budget, based on a promise which Jean Cretian had made at Kananaskus at the meeting of the G8 a year or two ago, Canada increased its foreign aid budget by 8%. Jean Cretian said it would be increased by 8% through to the year 2010 which interestly enough will bring us back to the level we had attained in 1985. Canada is roughly at 0.28 or there about. It's appalling low, compared to the average internationally which is significantly higher than that. If you look at the amount of money, the last year for which figures are available is 2000, but that's not bad. If you look at the amount of money, which Canada has devoted to International Health and Population Policies through its official development assistance, it amounts to 0.005 of gross national product. The only country in the Western world, which was below that, was Italy. Greece was at that level. The 20 other OECD countries were significantly higher than Canada. It's important for Canada not to pretend to self-righteousness about this kind of stuff. I happen to have a great deal of admiration and respect for the prime minister's initiatives on HIV and AIDs. I think Canada has done itself proud in a variety of ways. But I

also recognize that it was under the minister of finance, Paul Martin, when we began to slash our foreign aid budget in a way, which frankly undermined the reputation of Canada internationally. We are now desperately trying to compensate for those days. But all these countries who don't provide adequate official development assistance, have caused inevitably a great deal of grief in the developing world because of our cumulative negligence. Among the people who have commented on this most thoughtfully is Professor Jeffrey Sack, the world-renowned economist who until recently was attached to Harvard and until very, very recently moved to Columbia to head the Earth Institute. Jeffrey Sacks authored a fascinating commission study which I recommend to you, particularly the students that are gathered here called: The Macroeconomic Commission on Health, it flowed from the World Health Organization. What Jeffrey Sack did he was really fascinating. Essentially, he said, "If the world reached the 0.7 target, we would be having…$175 billion dollars to spend this year. $200 billion on foreign aid in 2007 instead of around $50 billion which is what we are now spending." He indicated that not only would that achieve the millennium goal of poverty reduction, but it would meet infant mortality rate reduction, maternal mortality rate reduction. It would put all of the girls who are out of school back into school. It would move some way toward gender equality. It would deal with water and sanitation, nutrition. It would make some progress of HIV and AIDS. It would above all create an environment where women and children's health were given extraordinary priority. But Jeffrey argued, that the disease burden, (that's what he called it), the disease burden of so many of these countries is so great, that you'll never get economic growth until you deal with the burden of disease. Up until now we have always thought about it in reverse. We have always made the assumption that if there is a great deal of economic growth in the economy that enough money will be generated to deal with the problems of human health and social welfare. Jeffrey said, "Nuts!" That paradigm has to be turned on its head. The burden of disease is so intense, it is so crippling to human functioning, that until you deal with the burden of disease, you will never, but never, get economic growth. On page 23 (if memory serves me) of his study he says as follows, "There are many reasons for the increase burden of disease on the poor. First the poor are much more susceptible to disease, because of lack of access to clean water and sanitation, safe housing, medical care, information about preventative behaviors and adequate nutrition. Second, the poor are much less likely to seek medical care even when it is urgently needed because of their greater distance from health providers, their lack of out of pocket resources needed to cover health outlays and their lack of knowledge of how to best respond to an episode of illness. Third as mentioned, out of pocket outlays for a serious illness can push them into a poverty trap from which they do not recover by forcing them into debt, or into the sale or mortgaging of productive assets such as land. A serious illness may plunge a household into prolonged impoverishment, extending even to the next generation, as children are forced from school and into the workforce. The entire argument of the macroeconomic commission of health is very simple. If we want to overcome poverty, which is what we're calling for, takes an appalling toll on women, if we want to introduce and element of economic and social equity without which there can be no social justice for children, then you have to, from the rest of the world, remove the debt, provide fair international trading regimen and provide social assistance. I remind you that article 74 of the rights of a child that every single child is entitled to the highest attainable standard of health. We are violating that convention which every single country in the world (save two) has ratified, every time we fail to honor our international obligations.

2. INFANT MORTALITY RATES

It is worth noting that the infant mortality rates in most developing world average 159 per 1,000 live births. Whereas in this country and other western countries, it's 6 per 1,000 live births. There are still 10-12 million preventable diseases for children every year. Children die at a rate of 30-32,000 a day from absolutely preventable diseases. It's totally irrational and heart breaking, that we should sacrifice millions of children every year for no reason what so ever except the inability of the world to intervene. They of course, are subject to acute respiratory infections, to severe malnutrition, which heightens every other opportunistic infection, or illness to which they may be subject. They also have malaria, tuberculosis, measles, tetanus, and diphtheria. All of these things take the lives of children and maintain the infant mortality rates excruciatingly high. It is so interestingly, forgive me if I am faintly academic at some of this exegesis, but I've always found it interesting when the convention on the rights of the child emerged, it emerged at a moment in time when the focus had been on what we generally called the "child survival revolution". Focusing strongly on the health dimensions and needs of children: thus the eradication of small pox, thus, the virtual eradication of polio. There were tremendous campaigns to deal with shoring up the health of children. When the convention on the rights of the child came into play it suddenly opened up a whole range of what we call "preventive issues for children", " protection issues for children". On to the agenda of the international community came child soldiers, child labor, child sexual exploitation, street children, disabled children, a whole range of youngsters whom the international community had not previously addressed; they were just part of conflict, part of refugee camps, part of internally displaced camps, they were part of the sexual trade. They were not seen as children to be protected. The world in a sense shifted ground over the last decade or so and began to concentrate on those kids. Until very recently the clamor has arisen today, you can't just deal with the protection issues. You have to go back to the child survival revolution and understand that the basic health imperatives of very young children are being sacrificed in this wide panoply of intervention. Every child is important. For heaven sakes, deal with them at every age and at every level...Children who are abducted and turned into child soldiers or sex slaves by a lunatic religious sect in Uganda have their rights and their health totally violated. Young girls who are taken out of schools to maintain a family that is suffering a terrible illness in order to maintain a family throw them into what we call transactional sex in order to bring some pennies into the home environment their health is terribly under stress and damage. The consequences for children in these difficult child protection areas and for their health are extreme. But all aspects of a child's health must be addressed. Canada has had some decent focus on some of these areas. Canada has always supported the use of oral rehydration salts in order to rehydrate kids who are suffering from diarrheal diseases. Canada has always supported the distribution of Vitamin A tablets in order to shore up the nutritional status of youngsters. What Canada needs to continue to do is to provide a very clear focus in order to overcome this pattern of huge preventable death.

3. MATERNAL MORTALITY

That is heartbreaking and mystifying in equal measure. I can remember when I was at UNICEF in the late 1990s, (forgive my being personal for a moment) and every year we would put out a state of the world's children report, and of course, you can't put out a report on children without putting out a report on the mothers. We realized that every single year, like methodical clockwork, between half a million and 600,000 women were loosing their lives in pregnancy and childbirth. There didn't seem to be any way to break the pattern. We discussed it time and time again. Despite all of the initiatives, which were then underway in the late 1990s, we couldn't break the pattern. Now personally, I believe, this is a manifestation of gender inequality. I've always believed that the absence of energetic initiatives, the absence of seeing this as a human predicament of the most extreme kind speaks to the general unwillingness of societies to respond to the needs of women. It is like an extension of the reluctance of men to relinquish power and authority and women are always given short shrift. Terrible things happen when that occurs. In the face of the pandemic gender inequality is fatal. In the face of maternal mortality, it means that only now, in the early part of the 21st century, are we beginning to take maternal mortality more and more seriously. I think everyone is agreed that skilled birth attendants and midwives, emergency obstetrical interventions where you can make them available, the consistent effort to educate mothers because the more they are educated the more they can forestall maternal mortality, making transportation available so that a woman who is in trouble can get to a facility which may be able to cope with that trouble if it hasn't been handled by, the one hopes, the skilled birth attendants on site. I remember one of the differences that occurred in the levels of maternal mortality in Bangladesh occurred when we were able to get cell phones into small communities, one cell phone per community. When a woman was in distress during childbirth or pregnancy, we were able to get word to the local health facility and summon some support. On the other hand, if they didn't have transportation, then the woman was lost. The United Nations Fund on Population activities is doing some quite remarkable work in the field of sexual and reproductive health. The kind of work, which deserves to be, supported everywhere and which the Bush administration in the United States has penalized (I think quite recklessly) by refusing to approve the $34 million dollars every year, which the congress has deemed to be for the UNFPA. The administration has turned it back. That's an attack on women. That would not happen if the money was designated for men. You don't have to even think about it for a moment to know that that is true. All of these aspects of training and birth attendants, and midwives and emergency intervention and transportation, and the sexual and reproductive health which has become more and more important for adolescents and youths, as the HIV/AIDS epidemic takes its toll – all this is (one hopes) the root to reducing maternal mortality. But to lose more than half a million women every year when it is utterly preventable, these are the things which should stir the passion in the souls of those of you who are going to enter the field of health. Because ultimately, with committed people we can break these strangle holds on women's health.

4. GIRLS' EDUCATION

Understanding the absolute importance of girls' education and understanding the pervasive discrimination against young girls, that exists in so many societies across the globe. Now, I want to remind you that we held an international conference in 1990 in JumChen Thailand, called "Education for All by the Year 2000". It was an international consensus that education, primary education should, as is stated in the conventions of rights of the child, universal and free. If we could get every single child into primary school we could for every additional grade that child took, would results in significant pluses in the future. Around health, or parenting, or simple knowledge, of skills of coping in life. There are between 115 and 130 million children of primary school going age out of school. Fully 60% of them or more are girls. Not only does it reflect again this constant discrimination against the girl child as they say. But it also reflects, the fact, that as families are making choices, it's the boy goes to school and it's the girl who does not. It also reflects the fact that when there is illness in the family, it is the girl who is taken out of the school to cope with sick and dying parents. It also reflects the fact, that in so many countries, particularly in Africa (where I spend so much of my time, so I am using it as a bench mark forgive me for not being sufficiently eclectic in the illustrations) but for many countries in Africa, there are still school fees – costs for books, costs for uniforms, costs for registration fees, costs for examination fees. They keep children out of school. They not only keep children at large out of school, they keep children who are orphaned by conflict. Children who are orphaned by the epidemic of HIV/AIDS. These kids can't get to school to have the sense of self worth. They can't get to school to deal with their peers and have a social context. They can' t get to school for the one meal they might have in a school feeding program. Who suffers most? The young girls always suffer most. If there is a fractional sum of money in the family, it will be male oriented in the majority of cases. Therefore the struggle to get girls into school is one of the great struggles that continues to exist. Of course it speaks directly to matters of health because the more schooling the young girl has, the more she is able to cope with the implications of parenting later on. It is also, I think, necessary for some country (and again I would love it to be Canada, I get this sense that I am levitating with romantic idealism about my own country), but I would love it if Canada were prepared to lead an international campaign for the abolition of school fees. With that must of course come some compensatory financing for the countries who abolish the school fees because they have become dependent on the school fees. If I may it is all so ironic. There didn't use to be school fees in Africa. Kids went to school free. Then along came the World Bank 1980's and 1990's, with what it called its "structural adjustment program" which was based on Reagan monetarisms. The consequence of providing loans to countries exacted from those countries certain conditions. One of the conditions was the imposition of user fees in health and in education. So suddenly, you had to charge for health. Suddenly you had to charge for education in order to get the loan from the international financial institutions. It was a punitive, repugnant policy. It was economically unsound. All these cerebral aristocrats, in the international financial institutions who are forever setting the agenda for the world and never fully understanding the implications. One of the most extraordinary ironies now, is that the World Bank rejects structural adjustment programs. It has said publicly, structural readjustment is dead. We have made a mistake. We no longer adhere to it. But of course, the consequences linger on in human terms. All these countries are saddled with the imposition of school fees and are relying on the revenue when it should never have happened. Therefore, we have to find some compensatory financing for them. It needs inspired political leadership from a country like Canada.

5. GENDER EQUALITY

I believe for what it is worth, that gender equality, the search for gender equality, is the single toughest struggle of them all. I think gender equality, to achieve it is much tougher than dealing with racial equality. I think that the imperviousness of male leadership to the struggles around women's rights has prejudiced the lives of woman everywhere on this planet. Sometimes of course, prejudiced it fatally. I have always accepted for what it is worth, a feminist analysis. I believe that feminism has made perhaps, the single greatest contribution to social justice of the last quarter century. The feminist analysis of power relationships between men and women seems to me to continue to constitute the most persuasive underpinning of what is happening to women throughout the world. I must say that in dealing with it on HIV/AIDs, it's unbelievably painful. Because the disproportionate vulnerability of women and the disproportionate susceptibility to the virus and the numbers who are infected, so much larger than the numbers of men, demonstrates to you what happens in health terms if gender inequality prevails. I think it is worth noting, that of the 25-30 million people living with the virus on the continent of Africa between the ages of 15-49, 58% are women. And if you narrow it to the 6-8million people living with the virus between the ages of 15-24, 75% are young women and girls. Those young women and girls have no capacity given the cultural realities to say, "No" to sexual overtures. Or to say, "Wear a condom." Or to say, "I want to negotiate safe sex." One of the things which is happening, which I could kick myself for not having intuited or understood before is that one of the most hazardous situations for women in many developing countries is to be married. Because the prevalence rates within marriages are actually higher than the prevalence rates in the surrounding community amongst individual women. The women think they are in a monogamous marriage and the virus is brought into the marriage by the partner. Usually, it is a young women and an older married partner. Therefore, the preventive mantras which we have fashioned are no longer applicable. Everybody thinks of ABC: A- abstinence. B-Be faithful. C-wear a condom. That's the applicable mantra, which was so effective in Uganda, to bring the prevalence rates down and is so effective in other countries. But it is not effective in marriage. We need a different prevention apparatus. Abstinence in marriage is neither possible, nor desirable. Being faithful is taken for granted. Wearing a condom is not possible to insist upon when the sexual relationships are so unequal. We need to think this through powerfully on behalf of women. Because in some kind of weird and twisted cuffcuesc way we are loosing huge numbers of women on the continent of Africa and beyond. It doesn't mean you don't work with men as well. But you recognize that it will take generations to change male sexual behavior. In the mean time we are loosing our women today. A virus which is driven by predatory male sexual behavior has to be stopped in its tracks. That means the women must be empowered. For Canada, it means that we have to continue our very considerable advocacy on behalf of gender imperatives written into every single program we advocate and written into every single international program. But that doesn't mean gender mainstreaming! If I have learned anything in the multilateral United Nations' environment – its that gender mainstreaming is a phrase I abhor! Once you think you have mainstreamed it into gender or gender is mainstreamed into a policy, it means you forget about it. It no longer becomes important. Indeed where women are concerned, you've got always to deal with it in a very special and affirmative way. Because just to mainstream it is to get rid of it from the public policy debate.

6. ENVIRONMENT PRESERVATION

Need I say more than to note what is happening in Haiti. Thousands of people who have died, likely cholera or other communicable diseases spreading as a result of the floods. The floods taking such desperate carnage because of course, there is barely a tree left on the entire island of Haiti. Because they have simply been destroyed in the process of trying to keep life together by the inhabitants. When you have absolutely no foliage, you have absolutely no vegetation to soak up the water, then you end up with a catastrophe that we are now witnessing. The need for the environment to be protected as an extension of health and recognizing that clean water and decent sanitation are a part of that, is very, very important. I want to tell you just with a mischievous smile that one of the projects that my little foundation is supporting is something called "Reach out Mbuya" which is a parish in the center of Uganda. Where they are doing treatment, and prevention and home based care and looking after orphans. My daughter runs the foundation, and I got this sudden desperate appeal from Sister Margareth Dunka who said, " We have to have a new latrine." I said, "But we are not really funding latrines." Sister Dunka said, "You don't understand!" The opportunistic infections induced by HIV as it proceeds toward full-blown AIDS and the state of diarrhea in the community requires a latrine. That is more important to us now than anything else because the sanitary disposal systems in the community are awful. So we huddled at this end. We discussed it with James Orbinski, that magnificent doctor that knows so much about the developing world who sits on our little board. We decided we should do it. Just a couple of months ago, I cut the ribbon on the Stephen Lewis latrine – in Reach out Mbuya in Uganda. I felt very good about it because I understood that the link to health was absolutely imperative.

7. HIV/AIDs

I want to just spend a moment on HIV/AIDs. Then we can have an exchange of questions and answer. Maybe we'll elaborate on it. What is important to understand about HIV and AIDS is apart from the terrible decimating consequences of the pandemic for countries, cities, communities, families, is that it is turning back every social, and economic index we have. All the social indices that I just discussed cannot be possibly be attained in the presence of the pandemic of HIV. All you have to do is look at life expectancy if you want an hallucinatory observation. Life expectancy which in most of the southern African countries Mozambique,

Angola, Botswana, South Africa, Zambia, Malawi, Zimbabwe, Swaziland, Lasutu, moving up the coast to Tanzania, Kenya, Uganda. Most life expectancy right now would be in the vicinity of 60 years or better without HIV and AIDS. It has dropped in 15 years, which is a pinprick historically, it has dropped in many countries to 38 or 39 years. It is expected in countries like Zambia that someone born in the next few years would have a life expectancy of between 32-35. It is as though we were catapulted back into the middle ages and just shows what happens when you loose your productive age groups. Women and children are the most vulnerable and the women carry the entire burden of care. We loose capacity. Death is omnibus, omnipresent, omni pervasive. Everywhere you go there is the reality of death. It is beyond one's capacity to convey. I can't tell you how many times I have met groups of lovely young women, they are always young, they are always in their 20's. They have their children in tow. They come up to me and say, "Mr. Lewis, what is going to happen to my children when I die?" Then they say, "You have drugs in your country, to keep people alive. Why can't we have drugs to keep our people alive?" There is no answer to that question. It just speaks to the grotesque disparity the unconscionable disparity between the developed and developing world

This speaks to the fact that we will send by the 2005, $260 billion dollars to fight wars in Iraq and Afghanistan. We can barely raise a smidgen of that to deal with the human condition. There are several things it seems to me that can be done, that we as a country can support. As budding health professional you might be interested in some of them.

#1. Right across the continent of Africa, and around the world, there are what we call prevention of Mother to Child transition programs: PMCTP. That is by enlarge the use of the drug naverapine to stop the passage of the virus during in the birthing process. A tablet given to the mother while giving birth, and a liquid equivalent to the infant within 48 hours thereafter, and you can reduce the transmission by over 50%. The problem is that the mother's always say, and it is perfectly understandable, "I'll do anything in the world to save my child, but what about me?" So under the eges of Columbia University and UNICEF and funds raised by a number of foundations led by Rockefeller, and an additional funds from USAID and CDC, they are now introducing what they called PMTCTplus. Where the plus represents treatment of the mother, treatment of the partner and treatment of any HIV positive children. The problem is that these models are very few in number and only tiny numbers of women get tested and go through the program where naveralbine or AZT can be introduced. I remember, I will never forget this, I was at the prevention of mother to child transmission clinic in Malago, the Malago hospital in Kampala,Uganda. As many doctors here can tell you, the measure in Africa which induced treatment is if your CD4 count drops below 200. For the first time ever, I was introduced to a woman whose CD4 count had been 1. Literally, two months later she was sitting infront of me, with her two kids playing around her feet. She was looking good. She had gained weight. She had gone back to work. It was absolutely amazing to see the transformation. In Africa, they call it the "Lazarus effect". It shows you what antiretroviral drugs can do. These antiretroviral drugs were generic, fixed dose combinations, 3 drugs in 1 tablet, a regimen of 2 tables per day and they were working miraculous wonders. One of the ways to reduce this overwhelming orphan population in Africa is to keep the mothers alive. That what this treated is attempting to do.

We also need (I think) a campaign where external countries can be helpful because of our legislative apparatus, against sexual violence and the enforcement of laws against sexual violence, and laws on property rights and inheritance rights, so the woman's position is not further compromised.

We obviously need to deal with the phenomena of female genital mutilation, which has caused so much agony across the continent and which some countries beginning to come to grips with, but need a great deal of support for.

One of the most exciting things that is happening, and I am glad to share this with you, as I bring these remarks to an end, is a scientific search for a microbiside. What the International Conference on AIDS at Bangkok showed in July, was that the search for a vaccine is still profoundly illusive. The international AIDS vaccine initiative is moving heaven and earth, to get there using biotech companies and major pharmaceutical and universities, in an effort to find a vaccine. But it still seems to be many years off alas. But a macroboside looks as though it might be discovered in the next 5-7 years. Most of the possibilities that are now in Phase 1 and Phase 2 testing are gels which the woman applies to herself and which prevents the transmission of the virus. Of course, the man need never know that the women has taken control of her own sexuality. But there is a very exciting development in the search of a discovery of of an intravaginal ring which will discharge medication over a 2-3 month period and will again give the women total control over her own sexuality. These efforts on behalf of microbosides suggest one of the most positive and optimistic aspects working on behalf of women. Canada has done itself proud, as I said at the outset, by committing a $100 million dollars to the World Health Orgainization in its coseneb to put 300 million people into treatment by then end of 2005. Canada has done itself proud by doubling its contribution next year to the global fund of AIDS, tuberculosis and malaria. Canada has not yet made a contribution to the International Partnership of Microbosides. That would be a further testament of our commitment, along with legislation to break patents and allow manufacture and export of generic antiretroviral drugs.

Finally there has developed internationally, a global coalition on Women and AIDS bringing together the activists in the Women's International Health community in particular, and the activitists in the Children's Health Community in particular, to mobilize around the millennium development goals and against the horrific consequence of the pandemic. I simply cannot convey in words, what is happening to the continent of Africa. I sometimes believe that some of the countries will not make it. I have been in the presence of the president of Botswana when he used the word "extermination" to describe what the country is fighting. I have been in the presence of the prime minister of Lasutu when he used the word "annihilation' to describe what the country is fighting. They are working heroically drawing on the tremendous sophistication and resilience of the grassroot particularly amongst women at the community level. But you can't have prevalence rates of 15,20,25,30, 35 40% in you 15-49 year old age group without taking an incomprehensible toll on the functioning of society. You loose infrastructure. You loose human capacity. We need your people. Then when it is all over, you are left indescribable number of orphans. The communities try to embrace the orphans. The communities are so poor they are pushed over the edge. So you have the phenomena everywhere evident of grandmother taking care of orphaned children. It violates all of the rhythms of life. The grandmother buries her own children. Then they look after their orphaned grandchildren. 10,12,15 children with the grandmother. Again, the women assuming the burden of care. When the grandmother dies, there is no-one coming up behind. So, you end up with this phenomenon of child headed households. We even have a word "sibling family" the older sibling looks after the rest of the kids in the family. You have large number of child headed households…. Continent where the age of the child leading the household is 8. You have to understand that there are no historical precedents for what is happening and the ruination of the health of a society taken in its broadest generic physical, emotional, psychological, is absolutely evisceration. There has been appalling criminal delinquency by western world up until now. Now there is some hope around treatment and resources. But we allowed more than 20 years to pass while people died in the millions unnecessarily. It has to come to an end. You are well placed in the future to make a contribution to that end.

In: Women's Health in the Majority World: Issues and Initiatives   ISBN1-1-60021-493-2
Eds: L. Elit and J. Chamberlain Froese, pp. 191-206   © 2007 Nova Science Publishers, Inc.

Chapter 11

WAR AND PEACE:
WOMEN'S AND CHILDREN'S HEALTH

Joanna Santa Barbara [1]

Department of Psychiatry, McMaster University, Hamilton, Ontario, Canada
Child psychiatrist, Hamilton
President of Physicians for Global Survival - Canada

ABSTRACT

In this chapter we will consider the impact of war on the health of women and children in both phases of the war system. Then we will turn to the efforts of women in ending specific wars, preventing war, and further, bringing about a peace system.

DEFINITIONS

War: Organized, persistent, mass, lethal violence mutually inflicted by two or more groups on each other [1].

War system: The organization of a society so as to be capable of waging war on another group at any time. This system is likely to be pervasive, affecting all aspects of society, for example, values, culture, taxation, education, entertainment, social expenditures. The war system will shape society whether in its 'hot phase' of active combat or its 'cool phase' of ongoing militarism, or readiness for combat, and will itself evolve to adapt to its social environment [2].

Peace: An attribute of a relationship between entities in which, at least, there is no harm being done by one to the other, and at most, the relationship is mutually beneficial and harmonious. Conflicts, which are inevitable, are resolved nonviolently.

Peace system: The organization of society (or other entity) so as to resolve conflicts within it, and between it and others without the use of violence, and so as to maintain mutually

---

[1] Corresponding author: Centre for Peace Studies, McMaster University, *joanna@web.ca*

beneficial and harmonious relationships with others. This will entail absence of structural violence (harm done by unequal, oppressive or exploitative relationships) as well as absence of direct violence. A peace system affects culture, values, education, entertainment, social expenditures, etc..

Health: A state of complete physical, mental and social well-being and not merely the absence of disease or infirmity [3].

WAR AND WOMEN'S HEALTH

War affects the health of women in the same ways it affects men, and then in further ways, peculiar to gender. Women are killed or injured when their villages are bombed, or their houses set on fire or grenades are thrown in their market. But in addition war can bring extremes of sexual violence to women and they can be affected in ways due to the role of women in caring for children and others in the community – the elderly, sick and injured.

Women combatants are subject to the same risks as men in war, and also to sexual violence from fellow combatants.

For noncombatants, the vast majority of war-affected women, the issue of sexual violence has, it would seem, always been an aspect of most (but not all) warfare, but has come into high relief in the last few decades.

Women as prime caregivers of children suffer unmeasured and immeasurable anguish in enduring the death of their children in war, their injuries, disabilities, starvation and ill-health. If they need to flee their dwelling places, as many millions do, they may be delayed and in danger as they attempt to protect their children. Sometimes mothers become separated from their children as they flee. They must try to care for children in the process of flight, during which, in fact, many deaths of children occur. Women may be pregnant and even give birth during flight. When they reach the 'temporary' camp, they must try to organize a household for their children in a tent or whatever is available, secure water, firewood and food, and protect their girls from the physical and sexual violence that pervades many such disrupted human aggregations. They must do all this while themselves suffering serious mental and physical illness.

In those camps of refugees and internally displaced people where settlement is far from temporary and may span a generation, women must endure the permanent truncation of their children's life chances, in terms of nutrition, health, education and subsequent employability.

Displacement causes many health problems to women and children. There are 32.1 million displaced people in the world, 80% of them women and children [4]. Most of them are in refugee camps. 12 million of them are displaced within their own country – 'internally displaced persons' or 'IDPs'. Whereas there are international agreements on care of refugees, there are none for IDPs; their plight is often grave. They must often organize their own sustenance.

Not all displaced people reach camps. Some subsist in forests for lengthy periods, with no access to outside aid. Health conditions for such populations may be very bad. In Congo in 2000, hundreds of thousands took to surviving in forests to escape rebels, militias and the Rwandan army [5]. Some war-affected women flee to cities, trying to avoid the privations and violence of camps. Without identification, they may be subject to police and other brutality, and many of them are homeless.

In refugee and IDP camps, women and girls are highly vulnerable. Even a male 'head of household' may not protect them. A man in Sierra Leone told interviewers: "If you do not have a wife or a sister or a daughter to offer the NGO workers, it is hard to have access to aid." [6] Women and girls must offer sex in exchange for survival requirements. Peacekeepers and humanitarian workers are sometimes the exploiters, as has been the case in Guinea, Liberia and Sierra Leone. The likelihood of high prevalence of 'sex for survival' practice is directly related to whether there is adequate provision of food to displaced people. In situations of high prevalence, such as Guinea, teen pregnancy may be as high as 50%, HIV/AIDS is rampant [7].

Domestic violence is also prevalent in refugee households. A man interviewed in Macedonia said, 'You need to understand. I am so stressed because of the war. It is inevitable that I beat my wife. That's just life.'[8] As an example of the extreme stresses that lead to wife-beating, a Congolese woman at a camp in Rwanda said, 'There can be conflict in the household. For instance, if I sell part of the camp rations to get food for a younger child, the husband will blame me if he is hungry, or he will take a young wife in the camp.' [9]

Displaced and other war-affected women and children are particularly vulnerable to trafficking, which is currently at a global level of some hundreds of thousands of persons a year. These are mainly women, and their destination is sexual slavery, domestic and factory labour [10].

In some countries it is marginalized minorities who are more vulnerable to displacement. In Colombia, for example, Colombians of African and Indigenous descent are over-represented in the internally displaced population [11].

DEATH OF WOMEN IN WAR

How do women die in war? First of all, they die from the direct violence of bombing, shelling, being caught in crossfire, being deliberately massacred in attacks on civilian settlements, and in landmine events. Few wars have been studied in ways that yield figures for female deaths.

Roberts and others sampled the Iraqi population in late 2004 to examine excess deaths in the 17 months after the US-UK invasion beginning early 2003. They found that in this period, in a population of 24 million, there were approximately 100,000 excess deaths, plus about 200.000 excess deaths from the city of Falluja, which had been subject to a particularly savage attack. Most of these deaths were due to violence from coalition forces, and the authors commented that such deaths particularly affected women and children [12].

Women die in child-birth in higher numbers during conditions of violent conflict [13]. This is likely to be due to their being less likely to give birth in hospital, and less likely to have access to a health practitioner. Giving birth during flight from home is particularly dangerous. War affects all three major barriers to women's seeking timely intervention to prevent maternal mortality: deciding to seek help, being able to get to help (over poor roads with inadequate methods of transport), and receiving sufficiently skilled help at a health station. It is not surprising then that countries hosting wars are more likely to have high maternal mortality rates [14].

Women die of infectious disease in war. This may be due to unsanitary conditions in camps, or to moving to an area where different pathogens find hosts in a less immune population. Death from AIDS may be a long-term outcome of rape, or of trading sexual favors for survival. These deaths may occur years after the acute phase of the war, and may not be counted in research into war deaths.

Threats to health are, of course, additive. Malaria, anemia and untreated blood loss in childbirth may add up to maternal death. During the period of comprehensive economic sanctions against Iraq, women who were weakened by malnutrition were more vulnerable to other health insults, such as loss of blood in childbirth.

Women in war zones die of conditions that would have been non-fatal in normal times. They succumb because of lack of health care.

INJURIES AND DISABILITIES IN WAR

Women may be injured in episodes of bombing and shelling. They may be attacked more personally in village routs such as in Darfur. In such episodes, injuries from rape are likely to feature. A very vicious form of injury is deliberate mutilation such as has been carried out in Sierra Leone by rebel groups. Amputation of limbs, breasts, and lips occur.

Women may be injured during and long after war by landmines. Women may be particularly at risk of landmine injuries in some circumstances, as it falls to them to get water, collect firewood and hoe fields in dangerous areas.

Landmine injuries deserve particular consideration because they continue, despite the international convention banning their use, to be a common cause of injury and disability to women in former war zones. There continue to be 15000-20000 new landmine injuries each year globally [15]. There is a distinct gender dimension to landmine injuries. Women predominantly have the responsibility to care for an injured family member. This may mean personal care duties for a crippled husband or child, as well as taking over farming duties or a paid job to sustain the family. An injured woman has a greatly reduced chance of marriage and child rearing, and of any further possibilities of education. Wheel chairs may be unusable in rural situations. Prostheses are costly; only a minority of amputees can afford them. The maimed family member may spend all her days in the boredom of her home, with greatly reduced social life.

The extreme proliferation of small arms and light weapons in zones of present and recent violent conflict has contributed greatly to the problems of women and children in those areas. Women are directly killed and injured, must deal with the deaths, injuries and disabilities of family members, are prone to suffer sexual violence and kidnapping for trafficking at gunpoint. Gangs armed with portable weapons may prevent access to relief supplies for women and their children[1].

ILLNESS IN WAR

In general, conditions created by war result in serious increases in prevalence of infectious diseases, frequently causing more deaths than direct violence. War conditions and the miserable living arrangements of displaced people provide fertile breeding grounds for HIV/AIDS, for malaria, and for epidemic water-borne illnesses such as cholera.

Economic need, the coercive power of young men with guns and the very high prevalence of HIV infection in some armies creates a lethal combination [17]. Incidence rates of AIDS have been found to parallel the rise and fall of violent conflict in areas, and geographically to correspond with the proximity of military establishments [18]. An association of war widows in Rwanda found that two-thirds of its members were HIV-positive [19]. Most cruelly, in some war and genocide conditions, such as Rwanda, deliberate infection with HIV has been an intentional strategy of ethnocide [20]. Malnutrition adds to the susceptibility of all elements of the population to illness.

Adding to this high-risk situation is the serious deficit in war of access to health care. War-time spending by states on armaments rather than human welfare, flight out of the country by health professionals, deliberate targeting by rebel groups of health facilities, difficulty with transport to what clinics exist, lack of money to pay for care and problems with health care for displaced and refugee people – these are some of the gross impediments to adequate health care in war. In East Timor, under war conditions, midwives lacked even soap to wash their hands before deliveries in childbirth [21]. In Palestinian Occupied Territories UNFPA reported that access issues continued to be an important barrier to women's utilization of appropriate reproductive health care, including family planning and obstetric care. Soldiers at checkpoints prevented ambulances and individuals on their way to health-care facilities from reaching the nearest hospital. Medical personnel were unable to reach their place of work regularly and distribution of medical supplies to rural areas was difficult. Delays have resulted in women delivering their babies while waiting to pass, which has led to maternal and infant deaths [22].

Even health care facilities under war conditions present risks such as transfusion with unscreened blood, procedures with contaminated instruments, contact with infected body fluids which may spread deadly infections.

REPRODUCTIVE HEALTH

Reproductive health for women in war zones presents particular problems [33]. Lack of contraceptive supplies adds to the burden of unwanted pregnancies in dangerous circumstances. United Nations Population Fund estimates that one in five women of reproductive age in displaced populations is likely to be pregnant [24].

Adolescent pregnancy and sexually transmitted disease increases in prevalence. 'In a crisis, the family support so vital to young people often collapses. A network that might have provided protection, help and information disintegrates, leaving young men and women more vulnerable than ever before. At the same time, youth traumatized by violence are particularly vulnerable to engaging in risky behavior as well as to sexual exploitation. Early pregnancy has serious implications for the health and well being of young girls, whose bodies have simply not developed enough to deliver safely and who are not mature enough to be parents' [25].

Providing prenatal care, safe childbirth and good postnatal care under war conditions is an enormous challenge, generally undertaken by the United Nations Population Fund and numerous nongovernmental agencies, in the absence of capacity of the state of residence of the population of concern. Care of the newborn under such conditions is an additional challenge. With the high rate of HIV/AIDS in pregnancy, transmission of the virus to newborn babies is a significant problem.

PSYCHOLOGICAL IMPACT OF WAR ON WOMEN

The acute and chronic stresses on women in war are extreme.

Five of Jeanette's seven children and her husband were murdered in the genocide. The youngest of the surviving daughters is HIV-positive. Jeanette has adopted two orphaned children. "When I wanted to tell the other children I have HIV, mine told me not to because of the shame. I haven't told the children about the youngest having HIV. It's difficult to tell a child of 16 that her young sister is affected by Aids. I try to be normal but I cry far from my children." [26]

Women suffer from depression, anxiety and post-traumatic stress disorder in the aftermath of the cumulative adverse experiences of war.

IMPACT OF WAR SYSTEM ON WOMEN

Most of what has been dealt with so far has to do with the impact on women of the acute phase of warfare, when shooting, bombing and flight from home are proceeding. The war system, however, continues in societies in the times between overt wars. Nation states maintain preparedness to go to war as a fundamental function of the state, and this has pervasive effects on the lives of women. The degree to which military institutions and values penetrate other social institutions may be referred to as militarization.

This will be expressed in the growth and resourcing of military institutions, and in military values. The predominating value inherent in the war system is that of prevailing by the use of coercive power. This will entail relationships that are hierarchical, involving dominance and submission. Compliance with the wishes of the dominating entity is valued. Disobedience is to be punished. It will also involve a construction of the world as comprising others who are either allies or enemies.

Many of these values overlap with those of patriarchal systems. Women may be thoroughly socialized in these values, although they affect women adversely in many ways.

States use a significant proportion of revenue, derived from taxation and other sources, to maintain armies and increasingly elaborate and expensive military equipment. Because this is often connected with maintaining a group in governing power, states will spend preferentially on these purposes, extracting finances from human welfare of the population [27]. Those in power will see military values as superseding all others, and will be prepared to override other values, such as fundamental human rights, refraining from torture and unfounded detention and imprisonment, observance of environmental standards, respect for indigenous land rights.

Militarism seeps into personal relationships and into institutions that should be far separated from the military. Burke, in an essay on 'Women and Militarism' observed, ' A US Inspector General's report on domestic violence concluded that military service is probably more conducive to violence at home than any other occupation because of the military's authoritarianism, its use of physical force in training and the stress created by frequent moves and separations. Military training encourages men to be aggressive and violent, and then asks them to keep these tendencies in check until they are "needed." It is no surprise that this violence spills over into domestic violence and rape.'[28] Research on family violence shows higher rates in military personnel in the US [29].

Militarism has long had a presence in the schooling of the young. Military-type drills and war-like battle cries have been common. Schools may formally be recruiting grounds for militaries. Sophisticated recruiting strategies are used by the military in US high schools. This pattern is growing in Canadian schools. Toronto District School Board and Toronto Catholic School Board have recently begun 'co-op' programmes with Canadian Armed Forces. Students get four high school credits and thousands of dollars in cash for participation in military training, including how to use machine guns [30]. This move was made without discussion with the school boards.

The presence of military bases has a strong association with the growth of prostitution in areas, especially if the region is poverty-stricken. Burke [31] describes the case of Subic Bay in the Philippines. This US military base is perhaps the most notorious example of the negative impact a base can have on the women of a community. Originally a small fishing village, Olongapo grew to have over 700 bars and clubs catering to the thousands of US marines and soldiers at Subic Bay. Although the Subic Bay base is now closed, when it was open, some estimates put the number of prostitutes serving it as high as 20 000. UN Peacekeepers, according to Burke, have also been implicated in prostitution. By the end of their operation in Cambodia in 1992, the number of prostitutes (many of them children) had risen from 6 000 to 20 000 because UN soldiers had created such a demand.

ACCESS TO HEALTH SERVICES

Women caught in war have reduced access to heath services for a number of reasons. In some wars, health services are deliberately targeted, as part of a war against a civilian population or to induce a population to vacate their territory. Even if there are health services, priority may be given to combatants, with women at the end of the queue. With many, or in some terrible cases, most women, having suffered rape, what health services remain may offer nothing for the health needs of such women. Reproductive health is poorly developed in many areas. Displaced people who had relied primarily on traditional healers may no longer have access to them, or to the traditional herbs and materials used. Community support, an essential resource in recovery from illness or injury, may have disappeared in the chaos of a refugee camp. Women in flight, or in IDP camps with no aid, or as urban refugees with no money will have no access at all to health services.

The group of experts commissioned to write the report for UNIFEM on 'Women, War and Peace' visited a desperate group of internally displaced people in Liberia. At a far corner of the camp, next to a ditch, a young mother of newborn twins sat in front of a makeshift hut of twigs and cloth. She looked about 17 years old and was sitting on a straw mat, with her family gathered around her. She had one tiny baby lying on her legs and another at her left breast. Her right breast was swollen to the size of a basketball. Her eyes teared up and she grimaced with pain when she touched it. Her husband explained that she had given birth to the twins a week before, just as they arrived in the camp; she now had a breast infection and her milk was contaminated. He said that (she had been told) not to feed with that breast, but when she didn't nurse, the breast got even more painful. "We need antibiotics, but we have no money and no way to get to the town even if we could buy medicine. There is no transport and they won't let us past the checkpoint." [32]

WAR AND CHILDREN'S HEALTH

Death of Children in War

Hundreds of thousands of children die in war each year [33]. They die of direct violence, epidemic illness caused by war, failure of health care systems in war, and of malnutrition. The Since the 2003 invasion of Iraq, infant mortality has increased from 29 to 57 deaths per 1000 live births. This change is typical of wars [34]. Comprehensive economic sanctions imposed on Iraq from 1990 to 2003 acted as a virtual siege on this trade-dependent nation, and resulted in the deaths of hundreds of thousands of children.

Injuries and Disabilities in War

As with adults, children suffer injuries in war, and these may result in permanent disabilities, such as loss of a limb, eye or neurological capacity. Rape of children is more likely to result in physical injury than in adults. Children are more vulnerable to landmine injuries and disabilities in a number of ways. Their exploratory nature exposes them to take more risks in the many areas of the world where landmines are sown in both rural and urban areas. Children are more likely to die as a result of a landmine injury. If they survive with loss of a limb, rehabilitation presents particular problems and costs, as prostheses, which are too expensive for many poor families, are quickly outgrown by those who have them. Injuries and disabilities interfere seriously with the schooling, social life and subsequent employment of children and teens. 8-10,000 children a year suffer death or injury from landmines [35]. In many countries disability means no option but begging as a livelihood [36].

Illness in War

As with other elements of the population, more children die of epidemic illness in war than of direct violence. Under–five-year-olds are particularly vulnerable to water-borne diarrheal illness, and there is significant fatality from this cause, especially among displaced people.

Malnutrution makes children even more vulnerable to infectious disease. In some cases, war-induced malnutrition worsens previous malnutrition due to poverty. Such long- term malnutrition may result in cognitive and social-emotional impairment, with little recovery on nutritional improvement [37].

Psychological Impact of War on Children

Children suffer many acute and chronic stresses during and after war. They may lose parents or siblings, their community, their home. They may suffer the horror of injury or loss of a body part, or of seeing others dead or injured around them. The extreme stresses and privations of flight or living in camps for the displaced are very hard indeed on children. Child soldiers live under brutal conditions for long periods. War orphans are an especially vulnerable population group.

Critics of Western systems of mental health classification say, in relation to the diagnosis of post-traumatic stress disorder that there is no 'post-' phase for people whose lives have been disrupted by war. The adverse experiences go on and on.

Special Problems of Girls and of Orphans

War and its grim companion HIV/AIDS causes many children to lose their parents to death or separation in the chaos of flight. In a study on unaccompanied girls in a camp in Guinea, researchers for the International Committee of the Red Cross/Red Crescent interviewed 22 girls between 14 and 19. Eleven had a child and four were pregnant. Information on reproductive health was available, but the girls had difficulty accessing it because of their children. They attached themselves to adult caregivers and often had their labour exploited and were physically abused. When food was short in the camp they often suffered greater privations with no family members to procure food and share with them. It was considered that these girls accepted sexual relations mainly in hope of finding a male protector [38].

Such girls are particularly vulnerable to being drawn into prostitution and kidnapped for trafficking. The fate of trafficked girls will be a slavery form of prostitution, domestic slavery or factory slavery [39].

Future Wars – Impact on Health

Humans have a difficult time recognizing and responding to phenomena that occur slowly by human time scales. There are three such phenomena occurring now, two of which are already causing wars, and the other of which can be expected to do so soon. These are human population growth, the peaking of petroleum production, and climate change. Wars caused by these phenomena will affect the whole population, of course, but will have differential effects on women and children as described above.

Human population, a fairly stable 10,000 – 500,000 for most of human history, has swung upwards extremely dramatically in the last several hundred years, especially since access to cheap fossil fuel energy increased food production potential. In some areas, competition of dense population for limited land and water has resulted in war. This may have been one of the contributing factors to the genocide in Rwanda. Competition for scarce water and land is recognized as one of the causes of the current ugly war in Darfur. As a cause of war, this factor can be expected to increase in importance as human population continues to grow and meanwhile, needed resources, damaged by human activity, continue to shrink. Most frightening, the expected mid-century population plateau at 10-11 million depends on rising standards of living, which may not occur because of the following factors to be discussed.

It is likely that we have reached global peak production of oil, and the gap between demand and supply will increasingly widen. The advancing oil scarcity has enormous implications for sudden shocks to the financial, social and political structures of all societies that depend on oil for energy. There is reason to think that there will be more violent political conflict in the future over access to and control of fossil fuels [40]. This is likely to involve major powers who want oil, control over oil, or control over the currency in which oil exchanges are made [41], as well as factions in oil-producing countries. Because of likely financial, social and political strains to all societies, those already stressed by social divisions will also be at risk of violent conflict.

We are seeing some of this now, with wars in Afghanistan and Iraq at least partly, perhaps mainly, to secure oil and gas supplies. There is also tension with Venezuela, Uzbekistan, Mindanao in the Philippines and in Nigeria, all fossil fuel producing areas. There is now and will be more political and military competition for dwindling oil and gas.

Inequities between rich and poor countries and between rich and poor in each country may increase; the poor are energy-poor. (ie no electric light). There is a risk of more human rights abuse (consider Nigeria), reversing development, reduction of environmental protection, increasing the sphere of control by governments. Achievement of the Millennium Development Goals is seriously threatened. There is possible increased risk of use of nuclear, chemical and biological weapons in this setting.

These problems will be exacerbated by the projected impacts of climate change. Global ecosystems are already showing negative impacts of global warming due to increased levels of carbon dioxide produced by human use of fossil fuels. Rising sea levels, increased desertification, violent weather patterns and unbalanced ecosystems will have direct impacts on human health, some effects mediated by epidemic illness. Populations will exceed their areas' 'carrying capacity', that is, the ability of a region to sustainably support a certain population. All of these effects are also likely to increase large-scale population movements to escape areas that can no longer support them, and to provoke violent political conflicts among the survivors.

Each of these projected causes of future wars involves food supplies. This circumstance impacts particularly on children, increasing mortality directly and through susceptibility to infectious diseases.

Remedying the Situation

Women insist on active engagement in all phases of work to improve the lives of war-affected women and children. For some aspects of intervention, it is reasonable to involve children too. We can consider responses at three levels:

1. Alleviating immediate suffering of war-affected women and children.
2. Building peace that takes into account the needs of women and children
3. Preventing more war

1. ALLEVIATING IMMEDIATE SUFFERING

A cardinal principle in remedying the suffering of war-affected women and children is their inclusion in discussions of how to help. As an example of application of gender sensitivity in working to improve the lives of people displaced by war, the Women's Commission for Refugee Women and Children carried out a study of the implications of women's role of cooking food in situations of displacement [42]. Gathering firewood is a task traditionally carried out by women and girls in many different cultures. For displaced people, it can be dangerous. Every day, millions of women in hundreds of camps risk rape, assault, theft, abduction, landmines injuries and even murder by simply seeking fuel to cook their families' meals. The Commission, by carefully studying the lives of the women concerned and consulting with them, was able to propose a number of remedies:

1. Provision of fuel as a humanitarian supply
2. Physical protection during firewood collection
3. Fuel efficient stoves. Besides protecting women from physical and sexual violence, this alternative also protects families from the eye and respiratory diseases produced by highly smoky inefficient stoves.
4. Alternative fuels such as solar energy

Each particular situation needs to have its own solution to the problem, worked out by women and men.

There are elements of international law that protect women and children in war [43]. International Humanitarian Law (laws devised to limit the harm of wars) and Human Rights Law (laws devised to limit the harm of governments to individuals, and applicable during both war and peace) are widely endorsed though often broken. International Humanitarian Law (IHL), embodied in the Geneva Conventions and additional protocols, specifies that all provisions apply to women without discrimination, that there is to be careful distinction between combatants and civilians in the conduct of war (frequently flouted in modern war), and that women must be treated with special consideration, particularly if they are pregnant or nursing. Infractions of IHL are war crimes.

Human Rights Law applies to many aspects of individuals' relationships with governments and their armed forces during war, such as the right to a state identity, the right of children to be reunited with their families.

Monitoring the implementation of IHL and human rights law during war is a major function of the International Red Cross/Red Crescent. Other human rights organizations play important roles as well. The International Criminal Court has been brought into existence to try war crimes. Women are watching carefully to see how the Court is used to uphold the rights of women. Breaking the impunity of rape in war will be an important accomplishment.

Many statements of guidelines have now been developed to recognize the special needs of women in war and situations of displacement. A definitive list of recommendations has been drawn up by the Independent Experts' Assessment on Women, War, Peace and Health [44]. These include 'Guidelines for Internal Displacement', 'Guiding Principles for Refugee Women', developed by the UN High commission on Refugees, and guidelines for many other aspects of women's and children's health under conditions of war and its aftermath.

2. BUILDING PEACE THAT TAKES INTO ACCOUNT THE NEEDS OF WOMEN

In dealing with specific wars, the incorporation of women at every phase of peace processes has been extremely important for the well-being of women, including providing foundations for the health of women and children. After a long advocacy struggle, this vital role of women was recognized in Security Council Resolution 1325, passed in 2000. This document recognizes the particularly adverse impact of war on women and "*Urges* Member States to ensure increased representation of women at all decision-making and international institutions and mechanisms for the prevention, management and resolution of conflict;

Encourages the Secretary-General to implement his strategic plan of action (A/49/587) calling for an increase in the participation of women at decision-making levels in conflict resolution and peace processes; ...*Calls* on all actors involved, when negotiating and implementing peace agreements, to adopt a gender perspective, including, *inter alia:* (a) The special needs of women and girls during repatriation and resettlement and for rehabilitation, reintegration and post-conflict reconstruction; (b) Measures that support local women's peace initiatives and indigenous processes for conflict resolution, and that involve women in all of the implementation mechanisms of the peace agreements; (c) Measures that ensure the protection of and respect for human rights of women and girls, particularly as they relate to the constitution, the electoral system, the police and the judiciary."

Implementation of these broad principles has begun, and there are significant achievements [45], but women in the peace movement feel aware of the importance of continual advocacy on these issues. It will be a long time before they are fully institutionalized.

An example of implementation is the application to the phase of movement between war and peace known as 'DDR' – disarmament, demobilization and reintegration, needs a focus on women combatants, who have frequently been left out of this process [46]. 'Women combatants, supporters and dependents have not equally benefited from services, cash incentives, health care, training, travel remittance, small business grants or housing support that flow to their male counterparts—males with guns—as part of DDR packages. The plea of a child combatant carrying her child in the demobilization camp in Liberia remains with me: "Don't forget me, I want to go to school." The terrible irony is that women and girls are not invisible to armed groups, who see them as essential, accessible—and often expendable—military assets. Yet having survived the devastating experiences of war as combatants, sexual captives or military "wives" and slave or willing labourers in the conflict period, these women and girls often become invisible when DDR planning begins.'

3. PREVENTING MORE WAR

Women are very far from being passive victims of war. At local, national and global levels, women are engaged in making peace in a variety of ways. This may range from war prevention strategies, to peacemaking dialogues, and after the ceasefire, to the long, arduous work of peacebuilding. Sometimes this is done in terms of actions from the health sector. Women health practitioners have been prominent in the violence prevention work against nuclear weapons and small arms, as carried out by International Physicians for the Prevention of Nuclear War.

There are many examples of women taking initiative of beginning a peace process, and drawing other segments of the population into the process as it develops [47]. Women demand an end to militarism, to the war-mongering of authoritarian leaders. The Women in Black of Belgrade, Serbia endured much persecution as they demonstrated silently week by week outside government offices, holding placards calling for peace and denouncing the government of Slobodan Milosevic. They were stoned, spat on, beaten and arrested. After they were internationally recognized with the Millennium Peace Prize from International Alert and UNIFEM, other women began to support them. Milosevic was eventually overthrown by the peaceful 'people power' of Serbian civil society.

Women in Black in Israel, symbolizing silent, determined dissent from Israeli government policy in the occupation of Palestinian territories, has maintained a similar weekly vigil for many years.

Somali women are accomplished in cross-clan peacemaking. In 2000 ninety-two women delegates from their clans attended the Somali National Peace Conference, representing themselves as a 'sixth clan' cutting across clan allegiances. They presented 'buranbur', special poetic singing by women, about the suffering of women and children in war. They asked for a female quota in the planned legislature. Against men's resistance, they secured 25 seats in a 245 seat assembly.

In response to Security Council Resolution 1325, many regional organizations, including the European Commission and the Organization of American States, have adopted resolutions calling for women to be included in peace processes. In addition, the African Union has adopted a Protocol requiring States Parties to ensure increased and effective representation and participation of women at all levels of decision-making. There are very few legislatures in the world that approach fair proportions of female representation, that is, half of legislators. Many think that militarism will decrease as the proportion of women legislators increases.

The only fully satisfying response to the extreme suffering of women and children in war is to work for the abolition of war. War is, after all, a primitive and unjust way to settle important conflicts between groups of people. It has the moral stature of two well-antlered bucks with horns locked in battle over access to a female. Humans have developed, and frequently use, far better ways to resolve or creatively transform their conflicts. The outcomes are generally more just, better supported and more sustainable than the outcomes of wars. Many groups in civil society, including groups of health practitioners and groups of women, work for the abolition of war. Physicians for Global survival – Canada, International Physicians for the Prevention of Nuclear War, the Peace through Health movement at several universities and Voice of Women for Peace are examples. In the work of such activists and of academics who can see the peace-health connexion lies the long-term hope of war-affected women and children.

REFERENCES

[1]   MacQueen, G. *Definition developed in lecture in Peace through Health course*, McMaster University, 06/01/23.

[2]   Rapaport, A. *Peace an Idea Whose Time Has Come*. Ann Arbor, USA: University of Michigan Press, 1992, chapter 9.

[3]   WHO. *Preamble to the Constitution of the World Health Organization as adopted by the International Health Conference*, New York, 19-22 June, 1946; signed on 22 July 1946 by the representatives of 61 States (Official Records of the World Health Organization, no. 2, p. 100) and entered into force on 7 April 1948.

[4]   United Nations. Women, Peace and Security: a study submitted by the Secretary-General pursuant to Security Council Resolution 1325. New York, 2002. *http://www.un.org/.womenwatch/daw/public/eWPS.pdf* (Accessed 06/05/31)

[5]   Rehn, E; Johnson-Sirleaf, E. Women, War and Peace. New York: UNIFEM; 2002, chapter 2. *http://www.unifem.org/attachments/products/214_chapter02.pdf*

[6]   *Ibid*

[7]   *Ibid*

[8]   *Ibid*

[9]   *Ibid*

[10] International Organization on Migration. New IOM figures on the global scale of trafficking. *Trafficking in Migrants: Quarterly Bulletin 23*, April 2001.

[11] Sanchez-Garzoli G. No refuge: Colombia's IDP protection vacuum. Refugees International June 3, 2003. *http://www.brookings.edu/views/gs_ri_colombia_2003 0603_page.htm* (Accessed 06/05/27)

[12] Roberts, L; Lafta, R; Garfield, R; Khudhairi, J; Burnham, G. Mortality before and after the 2003 invasion of Iraq: cluster sample survey. Lancet, 364(9448), 1857 *http://www.thelancet.com/journal/vol364/iss9445/full/llan.364.9445.early_online_publi cation.31137.1*

[13] Rehn, E; Johnson-Sirleaf, E. Women, War and Peace. New York: UNIFEM; 2002, chapter 3.   *http://www.womenwarpeace.org/issues/reprohealth/reprohealth.htm* (Accessed 06/05/30)

[14] *Ibid*

[15] Landmine Monitor Report 2005 *http://www.icbl.org/lm/2005/findings.html* (Accessed 06/05/30)

[16] Rehn, E; Johnson-Sirleaf, E. Women, War and Peace. New York: UNIFEM; 2002 *http://www.womenwarpeace.org/issues/smallarms/docs/salw_chapter.doc*

[17] UNAIDS. On the front Line: a review of policies and programmes to address AIDS among peacekeepers and uniformed services. New York: 2005. *http://data.unaids.org/UNAdocs/Report_SHR_OnFrontLine_18July05_en.pdf?preview =true* (Accessed 06/05/31)

[18] *Ibid*

[19] McGreal, C. A Pearl in Rwanda's Genocide Horror. Guardian Unlimited, 2001. *http://society.guardian.co.uk/christmasappeal/story/0,11321,612365,00.html* (Accessed 06/05/30)

[20] Rehn, E; Johnson-Sirleaf, E. Women, War and Peace. New York: UNIFEM, 2002. (Accessed 06/06/01)

[21] United Nations Population Fund. The Impact of Conflict on Women and Girls: a UNFPA Strategy for gnder mainstreaming in areas of conflict and reconciliation. Slovakia: UNFPA; 2002.

[22] *Ibid*

[23] Guy, S. The Impact of Conflict on Reproductive Health. In *http://www.unfpa.org/upload/lib_pub_file/46_filename_armedconflict_women.pdf*

[24] United Nations Population Fund *http://www.unfpa.org/upload/lib_pub_file/78_ filename_crisis_eng.pdf*

[25] Rehn, E; Johnson-Sirleaf, E. Women, War and Peace. New York: UNIFEM, 2002. *http://www.womenwarpeace.org/issues/reprohealth/reprohealth.htm* (Accessed 06/06/01)

[26] McGreal, C. A Pearl in Rwanda's Genocide Horror. Guardian Unlimited, 2001. *http://society.guardian.co.uk/christmasappeal/story/0,11321,612365,00.html* (Accessed 06/05/30)

[27] Ashford, M-W; Huet-Vaughn, Y. The Impact of War on women. In Levy, B; Sidel, V editors. *War and Public Health.* New York: Oxford University Press; 1997; p191.

[28] Burke, C. Women and Militarism *http://www.wilpf.int.ch/publications/ womenmilitarism.htm* Women's International League for Peace and Freedom

[29] Ashford, M-W; Huet-Vaughn, Y. The Impact of War on women. In Levy, B; Sidel, V editors. *War and Public Health.* New York: Oxford University Press; 1997; p192.

[30] Cash, A. Fast Times at Machine Gun High. NOW Magazine, May 26, 2006.

[31] Burke, C. Women and Militarism *http://www.wilpf.int.ch/publications/ womenmilitarism.htm* Women's International League for Peace and Freedom

[32] Rehn, E; Johnson-Sirleaf, E. Women, War and Peace. New York: UNIFEM, 2002. *http://www.womenwarpeace.org/issues/reprohealth/reprohealth.htm* (Accessed 06/06/01)

[33] Machel, G. The Impact of Armed Conflict on Children: Report of the Expert of the Secretary General of the United Nations. New York: United Nations, 1996. Available online *http://www.unicef.org/graca/a51-306_en.pdf*

[34] Roberts, L; Lafta, R; Garfield, R; Khudhairi, J; Burnham, G. Mortality before and after the 2003 invasion of Iraq: cluster sample survey. Lancet, 364(9448), 1857

http://www.thelancet.com/journal/vol364/iss9445/full/llan.364.9445.early_online_publi cation.31137.1

[35] UNICEF. Key Facts about Children and Landmines- *Profile of UNICEF*. JMA, 1999,3.

[36] UN Commission on Human Rights. *Contemporary Forms of Slavery: Report of working group. UN Document*: E/CN.4/Sub.2/2002/33, 17 June 2002.

[37] Djeddah, C; Shah, PM. *Report of the Study on the Nutritional Impact of Armed Conflict on Children.* Geneva: Food and Agriculture Organization of the United Nations; 1996.

[38] Holst-Roness, FT. Violence against girls in Africa during armed conflicts and crises. Addis-Ababa: International Committee of the Red Cross; May 2006. *http://www.icrc.org/Web/Eng/siteeng0.nsf/htmlall/violence-girls-conference-110506/ $File/International-Policy-Conference.pdf*

[39] Rehn, E; Johnson-Sirleaf, E. *Women, War and Peace*. New York: UNIFEM, 2002. chapter 1.

[40] Klare, M. *Blood and Oil: The Dangers and Consequnces of America's Growing Dependency on Imported Petroleum.* New York: Henry Holt and Company; 2004.

[41] Clark, WR. Petrodollar Warfare: Oil, Iraq and the future of the American Dollar. Canada: New Society; 2005.

[42] Patrick, E. Beyond Firewood: Fuel Alternatives and Protection Strategies for Displace Women and Girls. New York: Women's Commission for Refugee Women and Children, March 2006. *http://www.womenscommission.org/pdf/fuel.pdf*

[43] Lindsey, C. Women Facing War: ICRC study of the impact of armed conflict on women. *http://www.icrc.org/Web/Eng/siteeng0.nsf/htmlall/p0798/$File/ICRC_002_ 0798_EXEC_SUMM.PDF!Open* (Accessed 06/05/31)

[44] Rehn, E; Johnson-Sirleaf, E. Women, War and Peace. New York: UNIFEM, 2002 *http://www.womenwarpeace.org/issues/health/health.htm*

[45] Nakaya, S. Women and Gender Equality in Peacebuilding. In Keating, T; Knight, WA. *Building Sustainable Peace.* Calgary, Alberta, Canada: University of Alberta Press; 2004.

[46] Douglas, S; Hill, F. Getting it Right, doing it Right: Gender and Disarmament, Demobilization and Reintegration. New Tork: UN Development fund for Women (UNIFEM), 2004. *http://www.womenwarpeace.org/issues/ddr/gettingitright.pdf* (accessed 06/05/31)

[47] Rehn, E; Johnson-Sirleaf, E. Women, War and Peace. New York: UNIFEM, 2002 *http://www.womenwarpeace.org/issues/health/health.htm*

In: Women's Health in the Majority World: Issues and Initiatives   ISBN1-1-60021-493-2
Eds: L. Elit and J. Chamberlain Froese, pp. 207-219   © 2007 Nova Science Publishers, Inc.

ABSTRACTS

The International Women's and Children's Day has been held at McMaster University, Hamilton Canada annually each fall since 1999. The goal of the day is to increase our knowledge about the health-related challenges faced by women and children in developing countries and difficult places. Plenary speakers are from various disciplines and faculties in research, international policy, public health, situations of conflict, gender issues, international aid and disaster relief. Workshops are available to increase the opportunity for one-on-one interaction on a specific topic. Each year, research papers are accepted for presentation. An example of these abstracts are listed below. For further information about the IWCH symposium go to: http://intlhealth.med.utoronto.ca/IWCH%208th%20ANNUAL%20Symp osium%20brochure.doc

The International Women's Health (IWH) Group of McMaster University is a group of individuals who are committed to improving the health of women worldwide. Our three main emphases are: education, intervention and research. The IWH Group is committed to programs that have a holistic and effective influence on the lives of women worldwide. The Group is multidisciplinary and is a mixture of faculty, students and other interested individuals. Studentships sponsorships for work in an area of health in countries of low and middle income are provided by a grant from McMaster University and Organon. For further information see: http://www.iwch.org/symposium.htm

- **Title of Conference:** *Rebuilding Healthy Communities after Disaster and Displacement: Immigrant and Refugee Women and Children in Canada and Abroad. 8th Annual IWCH Symposium*
  Date: September 30, 2006
- **Title:** Meeting the Needs of Post-Tsunami Women Survivors in Rural Aceh
  Authors: ha-Redeye, Omar
  Location
  Objectives: To devise a better means of providing aid to post-tsunami women survivors in rural Aceh. Approaches taken by various governments and agencies in response to the Dec. 26, 2004 tsunami varied. Most did not employ principles of placing the needs of female survivors as a central focus. Banda Aceh was the primary destination for aid, and women in rural areas were largely ignored.
  Methods: By matching the culture and religion of the population, communication and performance was enhanced. Traditional routes of patriarchal authority were engaged and challenged to meet the needs of women. Interventions that considered

the preferences and outlooks of the local population were better received better by both recipients and stakeholders. Medical teams were integrated into the IDP camp and considered as part of the community. Rural women survivors were themselves able to identify their needs and allow outsiders to assist them in achieving these goals. Needs of the female population were at times specific and distinct from the general survivor population. Concrete strategies were implemented and specific programs were presented to meet these needs. Minimal control was administered in these programs to allow a self-directed application.

Summary: The appropriateness of western-style interventions should also be questioned. Some approaches were inappropriate, while others were even considered offensive. Interventions unsuitable to the area met considerable resistance and even had potential for volatile reactions from the community. Implementations of local faith-based psychosocial programs were preferred by clients due to familiarity and a higher level of confidence in outcomes.

Conclusions: Rights of women in the post-recovery period were often neglected by central governmental policies by citing political sensitivities. These violations are a concern for the entire international community under the Vienna Conference on Human Rights. Implementation of the Sphere minimum standards in the future will prevent such violations from occurring.

Presented at 3rd International Conference on the Impact of Global Issues on Women and Children, Dhaka, Bangladesh, Feb. 16, 2006

- **Title of Conference:** *Women and Children's Health during Unrest and Disaster-Facing Impossible Odds. 7th Annual IWCH Symposium*
  Date: September 24, 2005
- **Title:** Working in the Waste: an Exploration of Child Waste Picking in Phnom Penh, Cambodia
  Authors: Best, A., Chalin, C.
  Location:
  Objectives: The presence of child waste pickers on the streets of Phnom Penh, Cambodia can be attributed to a host of factors, all of which complexly interact to create a marginalized sub-population of thousands of vulnerable, working children. The children who work in the informal sector by handling the solid waste found on the streets and the dumpsites have specific health and social concerns. Organizations that work to address the needs of these children utilize different strategies when providing health and educational outreach.
  Methods: An eight-week study was undertaken in collaboration with a Cambodian outreach non-governmental organization, Community Sanitation and Recycling Organization (CSARO) that explored the background, educational status, work habits and challenges of child waste pickers in Phnom Penh. Included in the research was an impact study to identify how CSARO has improved the children's immediate conditions and their educational and future opportunities.
  Results: Results from the study indicate that children attempted to either balance school and work or were not attending school, that there were instances of domestic abuse as well as abuse in their working environment and that the children were exposed to a variety of health hazards. Children reported that they had learned a

variety of skills and had been positively impacted by CSARO. Recommendations on how to improve outreach were elicited by both CSARE employees and the children.

Conclusions: The interrelationships between socio-economic status, health status, educational status and street or dump work have thus placed Cambodian child waste pickers' in a significantly vulnerable environment. Organizations such as CSARO continue to work to address the immediate and long-term needs and rights of the child workers. Questions such as how organizations can remove working children from hazardous work, encourage families to support education and still provide basic street services to children in need still remain.

- **Title:** AOGIN-Asian Oceania Research on Genital Infection and Neoplasia
  Authors: Elit, L
  Location: McMaster University, Hamilton, Ontario, Canada
  Objectives: In 2000, there were 471,000 new cervical cancer cases and 233,0000 women died of this disease worldwide. Eighty percent of cervical cancer cases occur in the developing world. More than 50% of cervical cancer cases occur in the Asia-Pacific region.
  Methods: In an effort to control cervical cancer in the Asia-Pacific region, The Asian Oceania Research on Genital Infection and Neoplasia (AOGIN) was proposed.
  Results: AOGIN met in Sabah, Malaysia July 18-20, 2005. Present were over 200 delegates representing health care staff and researchers from 22 countries. The AOGIN constitution was accepted. The goals will be: 1. Collaboration and Research – the scientific committee will develop and encourage collaboration on clinical and basic research projects locally and internationally. 2. Scientific Exchange, Education and Training – AOCIN will be a forum for exchanging views and for cooperation between partners. 3. Information – AOGIN will be a teaching and information platform for physicians, patients and public authorities. 4. Surveys and Audits – A medical practice survey will be commissioned to assess practice effectiveness. This will be the basis for providing advice and recommendations to enhance good medical practice and improve financial management.
  Conclusions: This mandate was approved. An executive was elected and subcommittees formed. At the conference there were presentations from international experts in the field of cervical screening and novel technologies and preventive and theratpeutic HPV vaccines and their effectives. Several countries gave reports on either the status of cervical screening or education in their region. The next AOGIN meeting will be held in the Philippines in July 2006.

- **Title:** Obstetric Pathology of Poverty: Maternal Morbidity and Mortality Kep, Cambodia.
  Authors: Kalaichandran, Amitha
  Location: University of Toronto Centre for International Health
  Objectives: To study maternal morbidity and mortality in the province of Kep, Cambodia.
  Methods: A survey was carried out to examine maternal health in Krong Kep, using two questionnaires. The first questionnaire consisted of structured questions aimed at a sample of 300 pregnant or recently pregnant women in order to discern morbidity symptoms. The second questionnaire was a verbal autopsy where the best respondent was determined to answer questions regarding a recent maternal death in the area.

Results: For the morbidity portion of the study, 19% of the women interviewed reported symptoms of anemia during pregnancy. About 39% of those who had delivered reported having severe bleeding during labor. About 30% of the women suffered from postpartum hemorrhage. Women under the age of 20 and over the age of 35 were significantly less likely to suffer from postpartum hemorrhaging than women between 25 and 35. Five maternal deaths were recorded in this study. Since 523 births were documented in the district for the last year, the maternal mortality rate for the province is 956/100,000. The cause of death for one woman was unknown. The other women most likely suffered from infection, eclampsia, postpartum hemorrhage and antepartum hemorrhage.

Conclusions: Maternal mortality and morbidity in Cambodia continue to be a major health care issue in Cambodia. Many of the subjects interviewed never visited a health post during or after pregnancy, and most of the women prefer to consult a traditional birth attendant for delivery. Education and service-delivery is a necessary two-pronged method to improve maternal health. It is hoped that by improving health services for mothers, one can improve their health, as well as the well-being of their children. Universal access to health care is crucial for any MNCH programming to succeed.`

- **Title:** Community Obstetric Care in Boudhanath, Nepal: A 2-year retrospective analysis of in-hospital birthing center staffed by ANMs.
  Authors: Montgomery, A
  Location:
  Objectives: The Family Birthing Centre at the Stupa Sangha Hospital in Boudhanath, in the Kathmandu Valley, was established in February 2003. Since opening, the Auxillary Nurse Midwives (ANMs) have provided prenatal, intrapartum and postpartum care to women in the community. This retrospective study was undertaken to evaluate the outcomes of care provided by ANMs in the center.
  Methods: Charts of 172 women were reviewed and multiple outcome measures were evaluated.
  Results: Of the 172 women, 81 women delivered at the birth center, 83 did not return for delivery and 9 were still receiving prenatal care. Of the women who delivered, 11.6% received 4 or more prenatal visits, 39.2% received 0-3 prenatal visits, and for 44.2% there was no record of prenatal care in their chart. Of the women who delivered at the center, the induction rate was 1.2%, the augmentation rate was 13.5%, the episiotomy rate was 14.8% and the caesarean section rate and transfer to obstetric care rate was 0%. Upon discharge, no women received scheduled follow-up postpartum care. Firty-three per cent of women returned at 6-weeks postpartum to commence their newborn's vaccination series. In the intrapartum and immediate postpartum period, there were no significant maternal morbidities nor maternal or perinatal mortalities.
  Conclusions: The care provided by the ANMs in this small analysis demonstrates positive outcomes and identifies some areas that need improvement. Recommendations are made for screening for low-risk women, and implementing the World Health organization's recommendations for minimum standards of care.

- **Title:** Gender and HIV/AIDS in the Caribbean: An exploration of broad health system interventions to achieve primordial and primary prevention among girls and women.

Authors:

Location

Objectives: The purpose of this research is to explore gender-related risk for HIV/AIDS for girls and women in the Caribbean, primordial and primary prevention, including in partnership with other sectors of society.

Methods: The methods utilized for this research were two-fold, encompassing an extensive literature review and unstructured interviews with key informants to collect qualitative data. Research activities took place in Barbados, Trinidadand Tobago, and Canada. Key informants were selected by purposeful sampling, and individuals from various backgrounds, walks of life, education, employment sectors and experiences were sought. Interviews were conducted with individuals in the Caribbean and Caribbean religious workers. Ten key informants were interviewed and 8 provided verbal or written consent to use their comments in this research. Data analysis was coducted using content analysis which produced themes and categories, aided by the use of NVIVO computer software. The information from the key informants was interpreted in light of the literature and vice versa.

Results: A variety of risk factors were identified, many which are rooted in gender inequality: the gendered implications of civil conflict and poverty; Low self-esteem; Expectation that 'good' girls/women have low sexual knowledge; Multiple sex partners for males; Age-mixing or Trans-generational sex; Early sexual debut for girls; Lack of communication about sexuality. The following primordial and primary prevention strategies, that operate at the individual, community and society lever, were suggested: Transformative Approaches to address gender inequality; education; baseline of accessible services; truth-telling and no secrets from parents; limit exposure of young girls to men; fear; religion, obedience and accountability. Three important, and related, issues pertaining to the health system;s intervention in primordial and primary prevention emerged. First, a disturbing perception that health system interventions occur 'too late', after an individual already has HIV/AIDS. Second, the need for health system needs to partner with other sectors or society (ie., education, economic, legal, political, ect) in order to provide comprehensive gender-related prevention services. Third, the potential of the health system to be a 'neutral entry-point' by which individuals can both access health services directly, and be facilitated to access services from other sectors. In order to further explore this latter point, examples of such interventions from a variety of countries and contexts are provided.

Conclusions: Prevention strategies suggested by key informants, supplemented by literature, were of a wide variety, encompassing short-term and long-term strategies, at the individual and community level, directly probided by the health system and necessitating partnership with other sectors. Such a diverse range of strategies is necessary in order to address gender-related risk. HIV/AIDS are health conditions, and as such the involvement of the health system in prevention is key, yet one might question whether transformative approaches to address gender inequality extend beyond the boundaries of the health system. The health system can both directly provide certain prevention services, and for those that are provided by another sector, the health system may offer a neutral entry-point through which individuals can then be facilitated to access these services.

- **Title of Conference**: *Building a Stronger World Community: Both Locally and Internationally. 6th Annual IWCH Symposium*
  Date: September 24, 2004
- **Title:** Measuring New HIV-1 Infections in Sourthern India
  Authors: Paul Arora, Bridget Stirling, Robert Remis, Prabhat Jha
  Location: Centre for Global Health Research, St. Michael's Hospital, Toronto
  Objectives: India may soon have the largest number of HIV-1 infected people in the world. About 4.5 million people are currently infected. There are no reliable estimates of HIV-1 incidence (new infections). The literature suggests the epidemic in India is mainly driven by commercial sex work. Measurement of HIV-1 incidence is key to identifying the evolution of the epidemic, correlates of incident versus prevalent infections, and to monitor the success of control programs. Traditionally, incidence is measured through prospective cohort studies, which are difficult to implement. A "detuned" HIV-1 enzyme immunoassay identifies recently infected individuals using single serum samples. It uses the principle of increasing antibody levels: people positive to a very sensistive assay but negative for a less sensitive assay are characterized as recently infected.
  Methods: We will apply the detuned assay to measure HIV-1 incidence in hgh-risk populations in tamil nadu, India. We will study approximately 50,000 persons testing annually in 35 voluntary counseling and testing centers (VCTC). Aout 20-25% test HIV-positive. We will validate and apply a locally available detuned assay, and a previously validated incidence assay to 2,000 HIV-1 positive blood samples. Detailed questionnaire data on attendess will help assess possible selection biases and permit quantification of correlates of HIV-1 incidence.
  Conclusions: If successful, incidence testing will be extended to all VCTC sites in Tamil Nadu generating the first population-based estimates of HIV-1 incidence and its correlates. Such estimates of HIV-1 incidence would provide benefits for surveillance, planning of vaccine trials, and evaluating preventative measures. Incorporating a validated detuned assay into HIV-1 surveillance in southern India will provide a cost-effective way of estimating incidence in disproportionately affected groups, such as commercial sex workers, and generate the first large-scale estimates of incidence in south India where the HIV-1 epidemic is growing fastest.
- **Title:** Home visits as a method to increase utilization of professional maternity services in Yemen
  Authors: Chamberlain, J., Barbo, B..
  Location: McMaster University, Hamilton, Ontario, Canada and Sana'a Yemen
  Objectives: In the country to Yemem, only 22% of women utilize a skilled attendant for their delivery. This is a significant contributor to the high maternal mortality rate in Yemen (336 maternal deaths per 100,000 live births). There are many barriers including: 1a) availability of skilled attendants b) finances and c) distrust in the quality of services provided. This small study in Zaraga, Yemen was conducted to

see if home visits to pregnant mothers would augment the use of skilled attendants at delivery.

Methods: Female health care workers carried out prenatal visits for pregnant mothers (who were not attending a prenatal clinic) in their homes. All lived within a fifteen minute drive of the maternity center. The expectant mothers were asked whether they planned to deliver at the maternity center. The team encouraged them to deliver with a skilled attendant. A post partum visit was carried out to review the outcome and use of professional care during their delivery.

Results: As a result of the prenatal home visits, there was no significant increase in the number of women seeking professional care who initially planned not to deliver at the maternity center. Seventy five percent of those delivered did not plan to have a skilled attendant and did not use the maternity center at delivery. Twenty-five percent planned to use a skilled attendant and followed through with her plans. Only four (4) of the ten (10) pregnant mothers delivered by the end of the study. All delivered mothers had live babies and no maternal deaths.

Conclusions: The numbers in this study lack the power to show a significant difference and the study ended before all of the mothers were delivered. Larger studies are needed and a broader based approach including education of husbands about the importance of skilled attendants at birth. There may still be a lack of trust in the health care system within Yemen which prohibits pregnant mothers from utilizing the services especially when family finances are involved. Quality, free professional services are needed for all pregnant mothers in Yemen.

• **Title:** Assessment of two cervical screening methods in Mongolia: Cervical Cytology and Visual Inspection with Acetic Acid.

Authors: Baigal, G., Elit, L., Tan, J., Munkhtaivan, A.

Location: National Oncology Hospital, Ulaan Baator Mongolia, McMaster University Hospital, Hamilton, Canada, Royal Women's Hospital, Melbourne, Australia

Objectives: To evaluate the test parameters of VIA and cervical cytology in 3 Montaolian aimaks.

Methods: From 18Feb2002 to 12Dec2004, sexually active women, 30 years or older and who had never been screened, underwent cervical cytology and VIA in the aimak central hospital. All women with abnormal test results and 5% of women with normal results underwent colposcopy with or without biopsy.

Results: 2009 women underwent both tests. VIAA was abnormal in 254 (12.6%); half did not attend the colposcopy assessment. Pap smears showed ASCUS or worse in 3%; 2 patients with HSIL or worse did not return for colposcopy. Of those normals asked to attend colposcopy, 44$ attended. Using CIN 2 or higher disease on biopsy as the end point, the test parameters for VIA are sensitivity 82.9%, specificity 88.6%, PPV 12.2%, NPV 99.7%. The test parameters for Pap smear are sensitivity 88.6%, specificity 98.5%, PPV 51.7%, and NPV 99.8%.

Conclusions: VIA has acceptable test parameters for population based cervical screening in Mongolia. It is concerning that compliance with colposcopy was only 50%> Thus as process of immediate colposcopy or see and treat is required in this setting.

- **Title:** Health Care Beliefs in Mongolia
  Authors: Elit, L
  Location: McMaster University, Hamilton, Ontario
  Objectives: To determine the health care beliefs and practices in Mongolia
  Methods: A literature search was conducted using MEDLINE, CANCERLIT, GOOGLE, textbook sources at McMaster University using the text word: Mongolia, health care, newborn, women, immunization. Key informants from Mongolia who work within the health care system or in non-governmental relief agencies were contacted.
  Results: Health Care beliefes: Mongolians do not fully understand the health care principals or preservation of health and disease prevention. Sick care Practices: There is an increasing use of traditional medicines including certain foods (drinking urine), acupuncture and cupping. Endemic diseases include brucellosis (affecting nomads), bubonic plague and communicable diseases like diarrhea. Health team relations: the medical system is based on community feldschers (1,200 medical stations-> 29 Somons-> 12 sum hospitals -> 3 aimage hospital) and doctors supported by a hierarchy of hospitals and mobile emergency teams. Dominance Patterns: There is a profound respect for elders and the social fabric of the country is based in the family unit. Women are respected but have their unique role. Domestic violence is present.
  Conclusions: Mongolian health care practices are structured on the Russian hospital system with a mixture of oriental practice, folk treatment and western technology.
- **Title:** Empowering women for Better Health in Rural North India
  Authors: Henning, Paul, Gibson, Edna
  Location: Queen's University, Kingston, Chetna and Champak Community Health Projects, Duncan Hospital, Raxaul, East Champaran District, Bihar, India
  Objectives: The Chetna and Champak Community Health Projects operae in rural areas of east Champaran District, Bihar, India. Women's health status in this region is impactedupon by several interrelated factors including: illiteracy; gender discrimination; poor access to education, transportation, and health care; povertay; and other factors associated with women's low status. The projects have recently been shifted from a primarily health delivery role to a community empowerment focus in an attempt to facilitate sustainable development in the communities targeted, with an emphasis on facilitating women's empowerment.
  Methods: The projects focus on developing relationships with the villagers and forming groups helping to capacitate and mobilize them. The groups that are formed include village development committees, women's groups, adolescent girls' groups and goys' youth groups. Key components of the projects' vision that is achieved through the groups are: community organization; literacy promotion' capacity building' facilitating savings and low cost loans; encouraging microenterprise; facilitating access to health care; and developing networks with other service providers.
  Results: Good working relationships have been developed in 21 villages and 48 women's groups, 18 adolescent girls' groups, 13 boys' youth groups, and 10 village development committees are currently operational. Nineteen women's literacy groups have been formed with over 255 women and adolescent girls enrolled over the past year. Other project highlights include training programs for local birth

attendants and literacy teachers, health awareness programs and training sessions, formation of women's savings groups and micro-enterprise endeavours, and community initiated vaccination programs. Objective results such as percentage of women having safe deliveries, adequate access to primary health care, being functionally literate, having vocational sills, ect are currently being assessed.

Conclusions: The majority of communities targeted have been receptive to the health projects. Women are taking initiatives and working together to improve their health and social status.

First Prize

- **Title:** Relationship between Ocular morbidity, SEC and Health Attitudes in an urban South Indian Population

  Authors: Nikila C. Ravindran, Pradeep G. Paul, Hemamalini Arvind, Ronnie J. George, L. Vijaya, G. Kumaramanickavel, Catherine G. Chalin, David T. W. Wong.

  Location: Sankara Nethralaya Vision Research Foundation, Chennai, India; University of Toronto, Toronto, Canada.

  Objectives: India is estimated to have one-fourth of the world's visually impaired population with as many as 21 to 27 million persons with mild to moderate visual impairment in addition to the 9 million blind. Several studies have looked at trends between ocular morbidity and socioeconomic status (SES) in the Indian population, but have not related these to ocular health attitudes and practice.

  Methods: This study consisted of an analysis of 480 individuals 40 years of age or older who had been resident in the urban Chennai regions of Ashok Nagar and Anna Nagar for at least 6 months. Subjects were part of the Sankara Nethralaya Chennai Glaucoma Study (CGS) between June and August 2003. For each subject, visual impairment, SES and health attitudes and practice data were collected via detailed ophthalmic examination, standardized specially developed questionnaires and semi-structured interviews. Composite scores from the SES questionnaires were used to classify subjects into low (25th percentile or below), middle (25th - 75th percentile) and high (greater than 75th percentile) SES groups. Moderate visual impairment was defined as presenting visual acuity of 6/18 or worse, but better than 6/60 in the better eye. Severe visual impairment was defined as presenting visual acuity of worse than 6/60 in the better eye.

  Results: Of the 480 subjects, 12.2% (58) were visually impaired. Refractive error (50.8%) and cataract (36.5%) were the main causes of visual impairment. Moderate visual impairment was present at a higher percentage (67.3%) in women compared to men, and in those of low SES (46.9%) compared to those of middle and high SES. Positive attitudes towards ocular health and visits to an eye care professional were statistically associated with each other, and with increasing SES and education levels.

  Conclusions: Individuals of lower SES are more likely to be affected by moderate visual impairment, refractive error and cataracts and less likely to have a positive attitude towards ocular health or actually visit an eye care professional if needed. Public health programs should target lower SES groups, not only providing them with care for easily treatable causes of blindness, but also helping them understand the importance of ocular health.

- **Title:** Improving Pain Management In Obstetrics And Gynecology
  Authors: Watson MacDonell, Jo, R.N., M.Sc.N, I.B.C.L.C., McMahon, Eileen, R.N. B.Sc.N., M.N.
  Location: Perinatal and Gynaecology Program, Sunnybrook and Women's College Health Sciences Centre, Toronto, Ontario
  Objectives: A six-month rapid cycle improvement initiative was undertaken by staff in the Perinatal and Gynaecology Program at Sunnybrook and Women's College Health Sciences Centre. The Pain Collaborative was an organization wide initiative through which each program identified its own goals and strategies to improve pain management. Our aim was for women to experience decreased postpartum and post operative gynaecological pain through the introduction of a standardized approach to pain management.
  Methods: Pre- and post-intervention measures were collected. Several "Plan, Do, Study, Act" (PDSA) cycles were conducted in keeping with the rapid cycle improvement methodology. Evidence was used to guide the development of standardized postpartum and post operative orders, the creation of a pain assessment tool, an algorithm to guide nursing decision making to treat pain, and education strategies for staff. Collaborative team members received support from expert practitioners in the field, formal learning sessions and a web-based "bulletin board" provided information, support and networking opportunities.
  Results: Results of this initiative are promising and will be shared.
  Conclusions: Strategies for developing quality improvements through the creation of collaboratives will be shared.

- **Title of Conference:** *Making a Difference 5th Annual IWCH Symposium*
  Date: November 8, 2003
- **Title:** Revictimizing or Empowering? Preliminary Findings from Sexually Assaulted Women's Experiences of Undergoing a Medical Forensic Examination
  Authors: Dumont, Janice, Parnis, Deborah
  Location: Centre for Research in Women's Health, Toronto, Ontario, Trent University, Peterborough, Ontario
  Objectives: This study provides an account of the perspectives of women who have been sexually assaulted and who completed a sexual assault evidence kit at a hospital based sexual assault care centre for potential court use.
  Methods: Ongoing semi-structured, face-to-face interviews with sexually assaulted women who reported to Sexual Assault Care Centres (SACCs) across Ontario within the past six months.
  Results: The primary reason that women gave for presenting to a SACC was medical attention. Most found the decision to complete a sexual assault evidence kit difficult and refused to consent to certain examination components (e.g, blood extraction, pap smear). About half found the experience "revictimizing" and half "empowering"; the latter group stated that they believed having a kit completed would aid in convicting the assailant. Most felt that the medical care and counseling provided at SACCs was more important than the collection of medical evidence. Experiences with health staff

were overwhelmingly positive; examining nurses in particular were perceived as supportive and understanding.

Conclusions: Sexually assaulted women's health related concerns and overwhelmingly positive response to the general care provided by SACC staff reinforces the importance of collecting medical forensic evidence in the milieu of specialized hospital services. At the same time, certain tests and procedures within the forensic medical examination were found to be traumatizing and warrant reevaluation. Women should be advised that the collection of evidence may *not* help them see their assailant convicted. To fully account for women's perceptions of the empowering potential of completing a sexual assault evidence kit, follow-up interviews should be conducted in approximately one year's time, when the legal processing of cases is likely to be complete.

- **Title:** Victim Impact Statements: Do they help, hinder or harm? Preliminary findings on the views of social workers who work with women who have been sexually assaulted.

Authors: Janice Du Mont, Karen-Lee Miller

Location: Centre for Research in Women's Health, 790 Bay Street, 7th Floor, Toronto, Ontario

Objectives: This study examines the perspectives of hospital-based sexual assault care centre (SACC) social workers across Ontario concerning the therapeutic and legal influence of victim impact statements (VIS) prepared by women who have been sexually assaulted.

Methods: Ongoing semi-structured, qualitative interviews with SACC social workers (n=13) who assist female clients in the preparation and review of VIS for potential court use. Interviews have been transcribed verbatim and are being analyzed using the NUD*IST software program.

Results: Social workers indicated an overwhelming positive response by clients to the VIS in terms of "being able to tell their story" of the psychological, physical, familial and other impacts of the sexual assault. Some victim impact statements were prepared prior to, or in the absence of, an assailant's conviction suggesting that the utility of the VIS is not specific to its court use. However, social workers and clients generally found the court-approved format for the VIS limiting. It was felt that the VIS privileged physical injury over psychological sequelae, as well as victims who would be perceived by the courts their sentencing decisions.

Conclusions: Most social workers believed that clients found the VIS an "empowering" process when undertaken within a supportive therapeutic relationship. The potential therapeutic benefit of the VIS reinforces its importance even in the absence of the opportunity to present it to the court at the time of sentencing. However, the VIS may been seen as legitimating certain assaults and victims over others, a practice which may be harmful to women who do not conform to stereotypes concerning sexual assault.

- **Title:** A Qualitative Study of Sudanese Refugee Women and Their Mental Health
  Authors: Hajdukowski-Ahmed, M., Ploeg, J., Trolloppe,K., Carias, A., Wasuge, M., Henderson, K., Escobar, C., Bhaloo, S., King, K., Montan, C.
  Location: McMaster University, Settlement and Integration services Organisation (SISO) and the City of Hamilton Public Health and Community services

Objectives: Explore how mental health is understood, experienced and constructed by refugee women from Sudan. Assess their experience with formal services in the region. Explore the process of identity reconstruction, and the generation of informal support networks in the post-migration context.

Methods: Women 18 yr and older, who came as refugees and have been in Canada between 1 and 7 years. They came from Northern and Southern Sudan, belong to different cultures and religions (particularly Christian and Muslim, speaking Arabic or Nuer). They came from refugee camps of had to flee the country individually. Eight women participated in a focus group, which was followed by in-depth interviews of 3 participants from different regions and cultures, and an interview of one service provider.

Grounded theory. Continual, open (selecting categories of information), axial (interconnecting those categories) and selective (building a narrative that connects the categories) coding of collected data.

Results: Brief statements on main findings will be shared. They are the results of a collective analysis conducted by researchers and by a fourth year Arts and Science student, SB, who volunteered as a Research Assistant and wrote her thesis on the same topic. The analysis aims at answering the following questions: How is mental health understood by Sudanese women, from a gendered cultural perpective? How is it constructed from a gendered and Cultural perspective? In their terms, what were the pre-exilic mental health issues and healing strategies of refugee women in Sudan in their specific contexts? What/who has been helpful when they arrived? What mental health issues are they facing in Canada? What are their healing strategies? What existing services are they using? How has the refugee experience and the migration experience changed them as women? How do they perceive themselves now? What they feel they have achieved? What are their new goals and aspiration?

Conclusions: Limits of the study include a small sample size. More studies are needed with other groups of refugee women on how mental health is understood in their cultures.

- **Title:** Improving Pain Management in Obstetrics and Gynecology

  Authors: MacDonell, W., Mahon, E.

  Location: Perinatal and Gynecology Program, Sunnybrook and Women's College Health Sciences Centre, Toronto, Ontario

  Objectives: A six-month rapid cycle improvement initiative was undertaken by staff in the Perinatal and Gynecology Program at Sunnybrook and Women's College health Sciences Centre. The Pain Collaborative was an organization wide initiative through which each program identified its own goals and strategies to improve pain management. Our aim was for women to experience decreased postpartum and post-operative gynecological pain through the introduction of a standardized approach to pain management.

  Methods: Pre- and post-intervention measures were collected. Several "Plan, Do, Study, Act" (PDSA) cycles were conducted in keeping with the rapid cycle improvement methodology. Ebidence was used to guide the development of standardized postpartum and post operative orders, the creation of a pain assessment tool, an algorithm to guide nursing decision making to treat pain, and education strategies for staff. Collaborative team members received support from expert practitioners in the field, formal learning sessions and a web-based "bulletin board" provided information, support and networking opportunities.

Results: Results of this initiative are promising and will be shared.

Conclusions: Strategies for developing quality improvements through the creation of collaboratives will be shared.

- **Title of Conference:** *International Women's Health: Making a Difference 4th Annual IWCH Symposium*
  Date: November 8, 2002

- **Title of Conference:** *Health For Women In Developing Countries: A Right Defiled. 3rd Annual IWH Symposium*
  Date: November 9, 2001

- **Title of Conference:** *An International Crisis: Dying Moms and Shrinking Resources. 2nd Annual IWH Symposium*
  Date: October 20, 2000

- **Title of Conference:** *International Women's Health: What in the World is Happening? 1st Annual IWH Symposium*
  Date: October 29, 1999

INDEX

D

H

I

J

S